Getting Started in Research and Audit

Editor: Mary O'Kane

© The British Association, 1998.

ISBN 0 9529869 0 6

FOREWORD

Research and audit are the cornerstones of good clinical practice. We cannot ensure that our clinical practice is evidence based or effective if we do not gather supporting information. Many dietitians are, however, daunted by the idea of research and audit, thinking that it is the remit of academic departments of large teaching units. If dietitians feel they lack the necessary skills they will lack the confidence to embark on research projects.

This book addresses these problems by beginning at the beginning. It offers advice about how to define the question you wish to ask. It gives practical guidelines on how to write the protocol, what methodology you will need to use, and tackles the problem of statistical analysis. There are also useful sections on dissemination of your findings, where you might look for funding of your project and many other useful references.

This document is written for dietitians by dietitians. It recognises and addresses the problems that can often dissuade a practitioner from embarking on research and offers practical advice and support.

I wholeheartedly commend this publication to you, and hope that it will encourage each and every one of you to include research as an integral part of dietetic practice.

Alison M Dobson, MBA, S.R.D.
Honorary Chairman.

CONTRIBUTORS

Andrew Carver, B.Sc., S.R.D.
2 Meldrum Road, Kirkcaldy, Fife, KY25LE, Scotland.

Helen Crawley, Ph.D., S.R.D.
STORM, University of North London, Holloway Road, London, N7 8DB.

Jackie Edington, B.Sc., D. Phil., S.R.D.
Senior Clinical Nutrition Adviser, Abbott Laboratories Limited, Abbott House, Norden Road, Maidenhead, Berkshire, SL6 4XE.

Gary Frost, B.Sc. (Hons), Ph.D., S.R.D.
Head of Service, Nutrition and Dietetic Department, Hammersmith Hospital, Du Cane Road, London, W12 0HS.

Jacqueline Loach, B.Sc. (Hons), Ph.D., S.R.D.
Chief Community Dietitian, Bradford Hospitals Trust, Nutrition and Dietetic Services, St Luke's Hospital, Bradford, West Yorkshire, BD5 0NA.

Mary O'Kane, B.Sc. (Hons), S.R.D.
Chief Dietitian, Department of Nutrition and Dietetics, The General Infirmary, Great George Street, Leeds, West Yorkshire, LS1 3EX.

Liz Oxford, B.Sc. (Hons), M.Phil., S.R.D. Bristol.

Alan C Perkins, B.Sc., M.Sc.
"Goulds", Staverton, Totnes, Devon, TQ9 6AH.

Chris Rudd, S.R.D.
Dietetic Manager, Central Sheffield University Hospital NHS Trust, Royal Hallamshire, Glossop Road, Sheffield, S10 2JF.

Moira Taylor, Ph.D., S.R.D.
Lecturer in Nutrition and Dietetics, Department of Nutrition and Dietetics, Kings College London, Campden Hill Road, Campden, London, W8 7AH.

Rachel Thompson, B.Sc., Ph.D., S.R.D.
Senior Research Fellow in Public Health Nutrition,
The Wessex Institute for Health Research and Development, Level B, South Academic Block, Southampton General Hospital, Southampton, SO16 6YD.

Carolyn Watts,
Formerly Research Dietitian, Rank Department of Human Nutrition,
St Bartholomew's Hospital, London.

Claire Wright, B.Sc., M.Phil., S.R.D.
Department of Nutrition and Dietetics, Manchester Royal Infirmary,
Oxford Road, Manchester, M13 9LW.

ACKNOWLEDGEMENTS

When I "volunteered" to co-ordinate the update of "Getting Started in Research and Audit", little did I know how extensive a project it would be. The result has been a rewarding experience with so many members of the BDA contributing freely their Research and Audit experiences for the benefit of the profession.

In addition to the contributors, I would like to thank:

All the members who were involved in "brainstorming" or gave comments about the various draft sections.

Past members of Research Committee.

Pat Flanagan, Audit Officer.

Diane Talbot, Chairman, Research Committee.

Simon Forrester, BDA Information and Business Officer

The largest thank you of all must go to Pat Orbell of the Nutrition and Dietetic Department of the General Infirmary, Leeds, who has very patiently produced the various drafts.

Mary O'Kane, BSc. (Hons), S.R.D.
(Chairman, Research Committee 1992 - 1996)

CONTENTS

Introduction

INTRODUCTION

This new and revised edition of "Getting Started in Research and Audit" is designed to help dietitians working across all specialities and settings to do as the title suggests - get started in research and audit!

Why are audit and research important ?

Nearly thirty years ago, Mr Enoch Powell (1966) pointed out that some form of rationing was required in modern healthcare as demand was potentially infinite, whereas resources are, of course, limited. The necessity of rationalising healthcare entails a need to prioritise and to determine which treatments are the most effective in terms of both clinical efficacy and cost.

A key proposal in the White Paper "Working for Patients" (1989) was that healthcare professionals should make the best use of the available resources. The report recommends that clinical care should be audited to determine quality of service, outcome and value for money. Audit and Research are the main elements within a Clinical Effectiveness approach. The development of skills and practice in these areas is fundamental to the future credibility of the dietetic profession.

In November 1996 the White Paper "A Service with Ambitions" was published. Three of the key areas in this paper are: information, managing for quality and professional development. These are all pertinent areas to dietetic practice today, and are important components of The British Dietetic Association's (BDA) strategic intentions. The interface between these key areas and dietetic research and audit is complex, however the publication and dissemination of "Getting Started in Research and Audit" should facilitate enhanced practice in these areas. The BDA has recognised the importance of research and audit in a variety of key documents produced over the last 7 years, including Towards the 21st Century (1991), the Education and Training Strategy (1992) and in a number of briefing papers (1989, 1992, 1993). Essentially these documents argue that in order for the science of nutrition to advance all dietitians need to become more involved in research, evaluation and audit of dietetic intervention as part of their professional practice.

Most recently the "National Professional Standards for Dietitians Practising in Health Care" (1997) clearly describe the place of research within dietetic practice in order to ensure clinical effectiveness.

Why should you be involved in audit and research ?

- To achieve and maintain credibility of the dietetic profession.
- To defend decisions, policies, and actions on a scientific rather than intuitive basis.
- To improve both efficiency and effectiveness in dietetic practice.
- To identify models of "good practice".
- To justify the allocation of resources, demonstrate health benefits, improve service provision.
- To increase knowledge, skills and confidence of dietitians in their work.
- To obtain personal satisfaction and for personal development.

Why are some dietitians reluctant to become involved in research and audit projects ?

For many dietitians the terms "research" and "audit" can seem daunting - they shouldn't be! There can be a tendency to think that research and audit projects have to be planned on a grand scale. However many of the best projects address simple questions and hypotheses and yield very useful information, contributing to greater understanding on a subject and leading to change and improvement in professional practice. Remember, the very nature of our training encourages us to ask questions, to reason through facts and problems, and not to simply accept information at face value. All dietitians have the potential to be involved in research and audit projects. For example, "Do patients comply with dietary advice for a specific medical condition?" "How knowledgeable are school children about food and health?" "Is there a role for low fat diets in the treatment of gall stones?" and an audit question, "How many patients with diabetes fail to attend follow up appointments ?"

Some dietitians, while agreeing that research and audit are important, also feel that it takes up too much time. No one would deny that such projects do require an investment of time, but it should be an integral part of working hours. The benefits of good research and audit projects are being increasingly recognised by managers who need information for example, on the effectiveness of dietetic interventions, to justify the allocation of resources and improve service provision. It has to be accepted that some aspects, for example, writing papers will usually impinge on personal time. It is worth noting that an increasing number of dietetic posts now exist with a specific remit for research or audit however, managers must impress on purchasers the need for recognition of time to carry out research and audit.

Also most dietitians once they get involved in audit or research projects, find it such a rewarding experience that they get involved in further projects! Whether you are initiating a study yourself or becoming involved in one that has already been planned or started, this book will help you by guiding you through key considerations for success.

We wish you luck in getting started.

REFERENCES

The British Dietetic Association (1997) *National Professional Standards for Dietitians Practising in Health Care*. Birmingham: BDA.

Department of Health (1989) *Working for Patients*, London: HMSO.

NHS. *A Service With Ambitions*. The Stationery Office, London: HMSO. Dd 506 5193. 11/96.

Powell JE (1966) *A New Look at Medicine and Politics*. London: Pitman Medical.

The British Dietetic Association (1989) Briefing Paper Number 1, *Quality Assurance in the Workplace*. Birmingham: BDA.

The British Dietetic Association (1991) *Towards the 21st Century*. Birmingham: BDA.

The British Dietetic Association (1992) *Education and Training Strategy*. Birmingham: BDA.

The British Dietetic Association (1992) Briefing Paper Number 5, *Medical and Clinical Audit*. Birmingham: BDA.

The British Dietetic Association (1993) Briefing Paper Number 7, *Setting and Monitoring Standards in the Workplace*. Birmingham: BDA.

Clinical Audit

CLINICAL AUDIT

What is the difference between audit and research ?

Before going any further it is important to define the differences and similarities between audit and research. In practice, the line separating research and audit is often difficult to define. In general terms, research aims to test a hypothesis in order to increase the overall sum of knowledge, it could for example involve the evaluation of a new treatment or technique. Audit on the other hand is a systematic evaluation of current practice to identify areas which require improvement or review.

What are the links between audit and research ?

Audit and research are interrelated processes **(See Figure 1)**. Both are necessary to ensure that a quality service is delivered. Audit involves writing standards based on current information about practice. Standards are written using information derived from clinical research and consensus on good practice. In other words, audit and the writing of standards is the application of knowledge derived from quality research. Audit is an ongoing evaluation process, once standards have been written it is important that they are audited to determine whether they can be achieved. When it proves difficult or impossible to meet standards or achieve identified goals, it is necessary either to take steps in order to change current practice or, when this is not possible, to revise standards to an achievable level. Audit which identifies areas of practice which fall below the accepted standard may assist in highlighting areas of practice which require further research and development. **(See Table 1)**

What is clinical audit ?

Clinical Audit is defined as a systematic, critical analysis of the quality of clinical care, including the procedures used for diagnosis and treatment, the use of resources and the resulting outcome for the patient (HMSO 1989). **Medical audit** refers to audit carried out by doctors, whilst audit by the multidisciplinary team is generally referred to as **clinical audit**.

Similarities and Differences Between Research and Audit

Figure 1. BDA Research Commitee

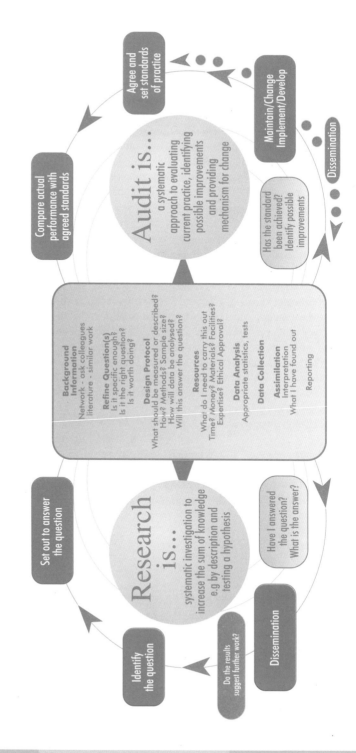

Page 8

What can audit measure ?

Traditionally the audit process should begin by writing standards of care and then evaluating whether these are achievable. However, deciding when to write a standard is something of a "chicken and egg" situation, as audit may involve the collection of baseline information on current practice, in order that realistic and achievable standards can be devised. Standards are usually broken into three elements; the structure, process and outcome. They can be tricky to write, but information on how to go about this has been well summarised in the BDA's Briefing Paper (BDA, 1992) on this topic. It is useful, also, to use local or national standards to determine how your practice compares with these, and if not why not, and what can you do about it? These could be incorporated in your own standards.

How do I carry out an audit ?

This section gives a brief overview of some of the key elements to consider in carrying out a clinical audit. Further information on audit methods is summarised in the BDA Briefing Paper (BDA, 1992) on this topic. For more detailed information the distance learning pack "Moving to Audit" (1995) designed specifically for the Professions Allied to Medicine is well worth obtaining. Elements of audit methodology are tackled elsewhere in this book, such as survey or questionnaire design, data management and statistical analysis.

To start you have to select your topic and then gather background information (see Defining the Question). Study design is important and is covered in the Writing a Protocol and Seeking Funding, Methodology and Statistics sections.

Your audit project may involve questionnaires (see Designing a Questionnaire). Once the study is completed, you must analyse your data and determine whether your standard has been achieved, identify any problem areas which need to be addressed and revise your practice or standard as appropriate. When you have collated your audit results sit down with your colleagues, look at the audit findings and literature in this field, and decide on the next steps which need to be taken. The absolute key to successful audit is to fully and critically complete this stage and be prepared to question current management, and change practice where necessary. Following this you should re-audit to see if improvements have been achieved, this is known as the "audit spiral", which currently aims to continually review practice in order to improve patient care. It is important to share your findings and conclusions (see Writing a Paper for Publication in a Journal, Abstracts and Posters and Dissemination sections).

Conclusion

Audit can often be seen as a dull waste of time and an unnecessary bureaucracy. However, a well thought out and positive approach to audit is an important component of ensuring that we keep up to date and offer a quality service (BDA 1989). This is not only a good thing for us as professionals, but most importantly it is good for the patient.

REFERENCES

British Dietetic Association (1989) Briefing Paper Number 1, *Quality Assurance in the Workplace*, Birmingham: BDA.

British Dietetic Association (1992) Briefing Paper Number 5, *Medical and Clinical Audit*, Birmingham: BDA.

Department of Health (1989) *Working for Patients*. London: HMSO.

Moving to Audit: An Education Package for Professions Allied to Medicine (1995) Postgraduate Office, Ninewells Hospital and Medical School, Dundee.

Table 1. CHECKLIST FOR THE STAGES IN AN AUDIT PROJECT

Stage		Questions to ask yourself
1.	Is there a problem in an area of current practice? **Define** the question that you wish to answer.	Why is practice suboptimal? Are there clinical standards? Who is going to benefit from the answer? To whom and how am I hoping to disseminate my results? (e.g. academic paper, managers).
2.	Gather **background information** relevant to your question.	Who might know of studies/a review article that will give me a way into existing literature? Which library is likely to have suitable articles? What would be suitable "terms" for a CD - ROM or Internet search of the literature?
3.	**Refine** your question in the light of the background information. Write your standards of care.	Has my question already been answered? Should my question have been partially answered, is it still worth pursuing perhaps from a slightly different angle? Can I clarify the situation if there is controversy within the literature? Are there local or national standards to compare current practice or do I need to write standards?
4.	Write the **protocol** for a study that will answer your question (include background to the question, methodology and method of data analysis).	Have I justified why this study needs to be done? How many subjects will I need? Can I use standards already tested by others? Will using different standards mean I can't compare my work with that already done? What data sheets will I use for collecting my data? Can I enter data into a databaseas I go along? Exactly which statistical tests will I use?
5.	**Cost** your study and apply for funding where necessary. Apply for **ethical approval** where necessary.	Will I need extra time or money to do this study? Who should I approach about this? Who can I check with to see if ethical approval is needed?
6.	**Collect** your data.	Is my data collection sheet working so that I can easily pick up on missed or inaccurate data points? How can I ensure missed data points are avoided.
7.	**Analyse** your data.	Am I keeping to my initial question or getting distracted by other questions that could be noted down and considered later?
8.	**Assimilate** your results.	Have I managed to answer my initial question? Have the standards been met? Why not, if not? What are the implications of my results. What other question/studies are suggested?
9.	**Disseminate** your results.	What is my time deadline? Would any other audience be suitable?

Table 2. CHECKLIST FOR THE STAGES IN A RESEARCH PROJECT

Stage		Questions to ask yourself
1.	Having "wondered what the answer might be to ....", clearly **define** the question that you wish to answer.	Am I absolutely sure that I have written down exactly the question that I am trying to answer, in the simplest way possible? Who is going to benefit from the answer? To whom and how am I hoping to disseminate my results? (e.g. academic paper, managers).
2.	Gather **background information** relevant to your question.	Who might know of studies/a review article that will give me a way into the existing literature? Which library is likely to have suitable articles? What would be suitable "terms" for a CD - ROM type search of the literature?
3.	**Refine** your question in the light of your background information.	Has my question already been answered? Should my question have been partially answered, is it still worth pursuing perhaps from a slightly different angle? Can I design a study that will clarify the situation if there is controversy within the literature?
4.	Write the **protocol** for a study that will answer your question (include background to the question, methodology and method of data analysis).	Have I justified why this study needs to be done? How many subjects will I need? Can I use methods already tested by others? Will using different methods mean I can't compare my work with that already done? What data sheets will I use for collecting my data? Can I enter my data into a database as I go along? Exactly which statistical tests will I use?
5.	**Cost** your study and apply for **funding** where necessary. Apply for **ethical approval** where necessary.	Will I need extra time or money to do this study? Who should I approach about this? Who can I check with to see whether ethical approval is needed?
6.	**Collect** your data.	Is my data collection sheet working so I can easily pick up on missed or inaccurate data points/ How can I ensure missed data points are avoided?
7.	**Analyse** your data.	Am I keeping to my initial question or getting distracted by other questions that could be noted down and considered later?
8.	**Assimilate** your results.	Have I managed to answer my initial question? Why not, if not? What are the implications of my results? What other questions/studies are suggested?
9.	**Disseminate** your results.	What is my time deadline? Would any other audience be suitable?

Remember! The most important stage is taking the small but vital step from "contemplating" to "starting". The road to research is paved with great intentions. Pursuing a "small" but important question that is within the scope of your situation, is nothing to be reticent about. It will certainly benefit the world far more than "contemplating" a potential Nobel prize that never gets past the back of an envelope!

Page 12

Defining the Question

DEFINING THE QUESTION

It is easy to take for granted the rationale behind the particular approach to a problem, however a patient or a student dietitian may raise some point which asks us to question our beliefs and justify our actions. You may feel that there is possibly an interesting project here, however it is worth establishing whether anyone has looked at these areas before. The flow diagram (Fig 2) shows the steps that you may take.

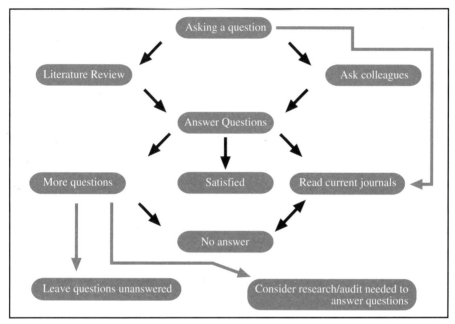

Figure 2. Defining the Question

ASKING THE QUESTION

First you must select your topic. A good project examines an area of current practice where there is felt to be a problem. It clarifies why practice is suboptimal, where care can be improved, and as a result should highlight changes which could help improve the quality of care delivered, make more effective use of resources or change clinical practice. Patients with Crohns disease, for example, have traditionally been treated with gut rest i.e. TPN or elemental diets. It has now been found that some patients do just as well on whole protein enteral feeds (Raouf et al, 1991).

Before you start, make sure you have clearly identified the question you are trying to answer and do not make the mistake of trying to answer large and non-specific topics like "Is dietary therapy effective?" A simple project may audit how many patients are weighed on admission to a particular surgical ward.

It is important to get some background information on your chosen topic. You should consider carrying out a literature search and liaise with your colleagues to see if a similar project has been completed already and to find out as much as you can to refine your question, (for checklist, see Table 2, page 12)

BACKGROUND INFORMATION

In order to answer your question, it is worth approaching colleagues both in and out of dietetics. Be aware that different people do have different views on the same subject for example, whether or not calcium intake affects the onset of osteoporosis.

Where to look for information

Within dietetics

- **Colleagues.**
- **Specialist BDA Groups provide** a great resource of information and may be able to place you in contact with someone in your locality.
- **The Research Committee of the BDA** consists of a group of individuals from various backgrounds including management, clinical, community, research and audit and will give guidance.
- **The Research Interest Group of the BDA.**
- **The BDA Research and Audit Register** is held at the BDA office and searches can be carried out for a nominal fee (available from early 1998).
- **Journal Clubs** in a department provide a useful forum for discussion of current literature.

Other sources of information

Contact and develop networks with others with similar interests or useful expertise.

- **Industry** - e.g. Marketing, research or training departments.
- **NHS** - e.g. Hospital/Community departments such as diabetes, gastroenterology, psychology, nursing. (They may run journal clubs which discuss relevant issues.)
- **Public Health** departments.
- **Health Promotion** departments.
- **Audit** departments.

- **Information Technology/Newsgroups/World Wide Web.**
- **Local education** establishments - e.g. university department of statistics, medicine, epidemiology etc.
- **Local service** providers e.g. environmental health, education department.

Find out about local, regional and national organisations that may be of use.

- **Sheffield Centre for Health and Related Research** (SCHARR).
  There may be similar resources in your area.
- **The King's Fund Organisation** holds a database of audit projects carried out by the Professions Allied to Medicine.
- **Health Education Authority**, other professional organisations.

Libraries

- **Medical Libraries.** Most teaching hospitals have large medical or post-graduate libraries for the staff which makes access to relevant databases and journals easier. If there is not a medical or post-graduate library in your locality you may be able to approach your colleagues in nursing, medicine or pharmacy.
- **Local Authority Libraries.** Larger ones often have good information departments with access to, for example, census data, local statistics, market research reports (e.g. Mintal/Gallup) and government, EU and international documentation (e.g. W.H.O.).
- **College Libraries.** If your research is not purely medical it may be that the local university or college libraries may have more appropriate literature. For instance psychology, social science, education and management journals may be stored in a university library rather than the medical library.
- **Current Abstracts.** Many journals e.g. Journal of Human Nutrition and Dietetics contain abstracts of relevant papers from several related journals. Various drug and nutrition companies have a helpline or provide booklets with reviews of current literature. The British Library Medical Information Centre at Boston Spa produces Medline Monthly Updates which contain current abstracts on medical subjects. Topics include Clinical Nutrition, Cystic Fibrosis, Eating Disorders, Inflammatory Bowel Disease and Obesity. There is an annual subscription fee.

Conducting a literature search

This may prove time-consuming and costly but is more efficient in the long term. If you are unaware of a good library near you, your local librarian will probably be able to tell you of your nearest medical/science library with the appropriate literature and whether or not you may use the facilities. You may require written permission first and may be allowed to photocopy articles rather than borrow them.

- **Get To Know Your Librarian And Remain On Friendly Terms!** His/her help may save you hours when trying to trace articles.
- **Abstracting Journals.** These are available in most disciplines. For example, a good medical library will have Index Medicus which will list medical papers under both the author's name and the subject. Other abstracting journals may be available in the library e.g. Nutrition Abstracts and Reviews.
- **Citation Indexes.** (available for Science and Social Science) may also be useful and can be found in college libraries.
- **Computerised Searches**. It may be possible to do computerised searches in various fields. One example is Medline which uses the Index Medicus data bank. The use of key words will help narrow your subject. Another example is BIDS (Bath Information and Data Services). There may be a charge for these services but previous reading will help you to be more specific and therefore waste less time and money on your search. A printout or floppy disc copy summarising the relevant paper details and often an abstract can be obtained. You may then decide that it is worth obtaining copies of what appear to be interesting papers. If the relevant journal is not in the library a copy of the paper can usually be obtained on inter-library loan for a fee.

Develop a filing system

As you build up your own research literature it is essential to develop a filing system which may be manual or stored on a personal computer. There are commercial packages available which will help you. (See BDA "Computer Software List"). This should be started as soon as possible and updated frequently. This usually involves writing out the authors name, title of the paper and journal (remembering to include the volume, year and page numbers). An example is:

Dunkeld Turnbull, J., Freeman, C.P.L., Barry, F., Annadale, A. (1987) *Physical and Psychological Characteristics of Five Male Bulimics. British Journal of Psychiatry* **50**, 25 - 29.

The reference for a book should also include the publishers, for example:

Garrow, J.S. (1981) *Treat Obesity Seriously*. Edinburgh: Churchill Livingstone.
You may wish to include key words or a short summary of the paper.

Do try to keep a photocopy of the reference paper so that you are not tempted to quote it from memory or use another person's interpretation.

In addition to including key words it may be helpful to code your papers and cards containing the titles e.g. blue for hypercholesterolaemia, yellow for diabetes and red for obesity so that an article looking at hyperlipidaemia in diabetes will have both yellow and blue stickers on it. When scanning through your files it may be easier to pick out relevant literature.

Although filing your references is a tedious procedure it certainly saves time in the future.

It may be overstating the obvious but it is worth keeping in mind your question. It is easy to get side tracked when doing literature searches by many papers which, although they may be of interest, do not help in answering your question. Keep your question as simple as possible because the most simple of questions will undoubtedly become more complex! Eventually your question may still remain unanswered.

REFINING THE QUESTION

Imagine the scenario, a medical colleague prescribes 1000 kcal diets for all his overweight osteoarthritic patients as he believes that weight loss is impossible on a higher calorie intake. You find, in practice, that the patients do not lose weight on an 1000 kcal diet and feel that the reason may be that compliance is difficult on such a low calorie intake. Your literature search reveals that obese people do in fact have a higher metabolic rate than lean people (Prentice et al, 1986), and also that people placed on 1000 kcal diets and strongly supervised always lose weight, (Garrow and Webster, 1989). You also find that a dietitian (Frost et al, 1991) has already carried out a study on overweight patients in an outpatient setting and found that those placed on an energy prescription 500 kcal less than their estimated energy expenditure lost significantly more weight than those placed on a 1000 kcal diet. It is thought that compliance is better with a more realistic dietary prescription. At this point, you may approach your medical colleague with the data and an outline of a possible protocol and suggest that you carry out a similar study on his patients who have osteoarthritis and are relatively inactive. You may decide to ask the question "Do overweight people with osteoarthritis lose more weight on a diet based on energy prescription rather than a 1000 kcal diet?"

REFERENCES

The British Dietetic Association (1993) Briefing paper Number 7. *Setting and Monitoring Standards in the Workplace*. Birmingham: BDA.

Frost, G., Master, K., King, C., Kelly. M., Flasan, V., Heavens, P., White, R., and Stanford, J. (1991). A new method of energy.prescription to improve weight loss. *Journal of Human Nutrition and Dietetics*, **4**, 369 - 373.

Garrow, J.S. and Webster, J.D. (1989) Effects of weight and metabolic rate of obese women on a 3.4 MJ (800kcal) diet. **Lancet, 1** 1429 - 1431.

Prentice, A.M., Black, A.E., Coward, W.A., Davis, H.L., Goldberg, G.R., Murgatroyd, P.R., Ashford, J., Sawyer, M., Whitehead, R.G. (1986) High levels of energy expenditure in obese women. *British Medical Journal*, **292**, 983 - 987.

Raouf, A.H., Hildrey, V., Daniel, J., Walker, R.J., Krasner, N., Elias, E., Rhodes, J.M. (1991). Enteral feeding as sole treatment for Crohn's disease: controlled trial of whole protein v. amino acid based feed and a case study of dietary challenge. *Gut*, **32**, 702 - 707.

The following references advise you on how to **critically appraise** a paper:

Crombie, I.K. (1996) *The Pocket Guide to Critical Appraisal: A Handbook for Health Care Professionals*. London: BMJ Publishing Group

Fowkes, F.G.R. and Fulton, P.M. (1991) Critical appraisal of published research: introductory guide lines. *British Medical Journal* **302** 1136 - 40.

Greenhalgh, T. (1997) *How to Read a Paper*, London: BMJ Publishing Group.

ADDRESSES

The British Library Medical Information Centre, Boston Spa, Wetherby, W. Yorks, LS23 7BQ. Tel No 01937 546039.

King's Fund Organisation, 126 Albert Street, London. W1 7NF. Tel 0171 267 6111.

Health Education Authority, Trevelyan House, 30 Great Peter Street, London SW1P 2HW

General HEA Information, Tel 0171 413 1995. Publications, Tel 0171 413 1986.

OTHER USEFUL ADDRESSES

NHS Centre for Reviews and Dissemination
The NHS Centre for Reviews and Dissemination (CRD) was established in January 1994 to provide the NHS with important information on the effectiveness of treatments and the delivery and organisation of health care. It aims to help promote research based practice in the NHS by offering rigorous and systematic reviews as selected topics, a data base of good quality reviews and a dissemination service. The CRD is the sibling organisation of the UK Cochrane Centre.

Address: NHS Centre for Reviews and Dissemination
             University of York, York YO1 5DD
             E-Mail: revolis@york.ac.uk

UK Cochrane Centre

The Cochrane Collaboration is an international network of individuals and institutions committed to preparing, maintaining and disseminating systematic reviews of the effects of health care.

Address: UK Cochrane Centre, NHS R&D Programme, Summertown Pavilion,
            Middle Way, Oxford OX2 7LG
            Tel 01865 516 300. Fax 01865 516 311
            E-Mail: general@cochrane.co.uk

Nuffield Institute for Health

This is based at the University of Leeds and is internationally known for its excellence as an academic institution in the fields of health and social policy and management practice. It has recently broadened its base to include public health, health services research and community care research.

Health Management Information Service (HELMIS) comprises a broad range of services which provide subscribers with access to the literature on health and social care management and policy in the UK and internationally. HELMIS is based in the Information Resource Centre of the Nuffield Institute for Health. For further information about HELMIS Services contact:

HELMIS Manager, Nuffield Institute for Health, Information Resource Centre, Leeds University Library, 71 - 75 Clarendon Road, Leeds LS2 9PL. Tel: 0113 233 6974. Fax: 0113 246 0899. E-Mail: d.a.unsworth@leeds.ac.uk

For further information about any aspect of the Institute's work, contact the Information and Admissions Office at:
The Nuffield Institute. Tel: 0113 233 6633. Fax: 0113 246 0899. E-Mail: v.p.sercombe@leeds.ac.uk

Writing a Protocol and Seeking Funding

WRITING A PROTOCOL AND SEEKING FUNDING

Once a hypothesis or research question has been developed, the next stage is writing the research protocol. This is a working document giving details of your project, exactly how it is to be carried out or implemented and who is involved.

Why write a protocol ?

Research ideas should never be lost. As soon as the inspiration hits you, put pen to paper. A protocol should crystallise your ideas, methods and study design. It is essential to write a protocol, even if you are not seeking funding. A written protocol allows others to comment on your ideas, so seek out people with experience in research methods for comments. Most experienced researchers spend many hours over this and write several, so don't be put off if it takes time to reach the final version! The first or second draft should be for your benefit, colleagues, and collaborators for comments before any submission to managers, ethical committees or funding bodies.

If the intention is to submit the protocol for consideration by a funding and ethical committee then you need to keep them in mind when you write. Once your study is underway, your protocol becomes a source of reference allowing for consistency of approach. It is also a good base for writing up and presentation of work at the end of the project.

Applying for funding

Many useful audit and research projects can be carried out without the need for additional funding. There is money available at many levels, and if you have a good project and are willing to invest your time in seeking out funding, you may well be successful. Grant giving bodies usually have very specific remits for funding and it is therefore important only to apply to appropriate funding bodies. Most funds are available for actual research projects, but if you need funds to write up research, to complete a project or to do a pilot study there may be specific funds available to you.

WRITING THE PROTOCOL

Protocol writing is an act of persuasive communication. You should aim to present a clear, accurate picture of the work you want funded to convince reviewers that the proposal is:

- Methodologically sound and likely to succeed.
- Worthwhile in terms of potential outcome.
- In the hands of a well-qualified and experienced principal investigator, (if it is a large scale research project), who will ensure it is completed.
- Supported by your manager if a smaller audit/research project.
- Appropriate for support by the funding body.

Protocol

Wording should be kept simple, so it is easily understood by all readers. Each organisation will have its own guidelines for protocols and these need to be carefully followed. In general, protocols will include:

A covering letter

This may be needed if applying for funding. Addressed to the appropriate person, the letter should be brief, noting the attachment of the protocol, number of copies sent, and should specify which type of grant or grant initiative the application is relevant to.

Title page

The project title often determines where the protocol will be sent for review, so write this with care, only using keywords of relevance and importance to your project. For example, "A seven day dietary assessment followed by an extensive diabetic education programme and reassessment in patients with diabetes" would read better as "Dietary intake of patients with diabetes before and after dietetic advice".

Other information for the title page generally includes the following:

*   Names of those applying and their qualifications.
*   The address where the work will be carried out.
*   The project timescale.
*   A summary of the gross amount of funds requested.

Abstract or summary (see section on Abstracts and Posters)

Always write this last. It is a complete overview of the project including the research objectives, methodologies, timetable and requested budget. It is usually limited to about 200 - 300 words.

Aims of the project

This section states what should be accomplished.

Introduction and background

This section outlines other work done in your area and gives background information on the significance of the study area. It is also a chance for you to show that you are up to date in your subject area, have kept abreast of relevant publications and theories and can scientifically review your topic. Your introduction should aim to illustrate that the study or audit you propose is a logical extension to earlier work completed or opens up an important new area - but don't make it too long.

Method section (see sections on Methodology and Statistics)

This is the most crucial section of the proposal. Make it clear which methods need to be developed during the research and how. Indicate clearly who will be doing the work and what experience they have e.g. "a state registered dietitian with four years experience in lipid clinic work". Always use recent published references if available.

The social sciences use many qualitative research methods which may be useful for dietitians - particularly those working in community nutrition. Present the value and limitations of those techniques chosen.

Timetable

Most proposals require a timetable for completion of work, specifying the time allocated to different stages of the study. Provide the best estimates you can for the various stages of the project and allow additional time for slippage e.g. holidays, sickness, etc. Even the most unexpected events can happen, and hold up a project e.g. faulty or unavailable equipment, transport or postal problems!

Resources

Even those planning to carry out unfunded projects should carefully consider the resource implications. A researcher who has not got an established track record of research should keep budget requests conservative. Preparing the budget will invariably involve liaison with finance staff at your place of work, and costs will vary tremendously depending on the project type and the amount of overhead your establishment of work demands. Briefly, resources which may be required in a research and audit project may include:

- **Personnel:** often amounts to 80% of the budget requested. Allowances for tax, national insurance and pay awards need to be made on top of establishing the appropriate pay scales for each staff member involved, and the percentage of their time that will be allocated to the project. When not applying for funding, determine how much release time is needed and negotiate this with your manager. Good record keeping may allow a project to be carried out without a substantial time commitment.

- **Equipment, materials and supplies:** the amount of money allowed for capital expenditure will vary, but costing for consumables should be made with care, and allow for price increases e.g. computers, dietary assessment programs, data collection forms, etc.
- **Subject recruitment:** this may involve paying subjects' expenses, for example, providing food/drink/medicine etc. and actual recruitment costs in some cases.
- **Travel:** this will vary enormously and costs will depend on the type of travel and frequency.
- **Other expenses:** these include computer time, telephones, stationary and postage, photocopying, use of the library, use of secretarial services, attendance at conferences or meetings etc.
- **Overheads:** most establishments expect an add-on cost of anything between 10 - 40% on all projects. Some research grants specify a maximum allowance, some allow overheads on personnel costs only, others refuse to pay overheads at all. Always discuss this with your finance director.

Justification should be provided for each budget item. If you include costs for a personal computer for example, you should be able to justify the need for such an item for your project alone. Many grant bodies expect that equipment such as computers should be provided by your place of work. It is important to prepare a realistic budget. If you under-estimate costs you may have problems completing the project; over-estimate and your project may compare unfavourably with others submitted.

Curriculum Vitae

It is usual for a brief C.V. of research workers involved to be included. Try and give the impression, from your experience, that you are professional, have the appropriate skills and are competent.

Other information

You may be asked to provide information on other areas such as whether other funding is available for the project; whether you have submitted your request to other bodies; how much internal support you will be given etc.

References and Appendices

You will of course need to provide full references for studies described in your introduction and methods sections. You may wish to include additional data in appendices.

SEEKING FUNDING

General tips for grant applications

- Find out as much as you can about the remit for funds for any organisation you apply to. Don't apply if your study does not fit their criteria. You can ask for lists of recently funded areas which may help to pinpoint their specific areas of interest.
- It is a good idea to telephone an organisation before sending an application, they will often be happy to discuss your project and will tell you if they would be interested in receiving an application.
- Ask anyone who has previously applied to an organisation for advice, it often helps to know who the reviewers are likely to be; networking can be useful here.
- Follow the application instructions to the letter. If an organisation receives many applications the first sift often means that those who have ignored the instructions are removed before review.
- Good presentation is essential. Remember your application will probably be photocopied many times, so it needs to be typed, well spaced, clear and easy to read.
- Check spelling and grammar carefully.
- Send your proposal to experienced colleagues for review before you submit. Don't leave application preparation so close to the deadline that you do not have time to allow for internal comments and corrections.
- Keep copies of all your applications and make sure that anyone in your organisation who should be informed about your application is sent a copy.
- Follow up any rejections as there may be a simple reason for a failed application which can be sorted out for a second attempt. For example, you may find the competition for funding for some awards is seasonally variable, and an application later in the year may have more chance of success.
- You may have to write a lot of applications before you have success. Don't lose heart, it is the same for even very experienced researchers.
- Check the freedom to publish the results.

INVESTIGATE THE FOLLOWING SOURCES

The British Dietetic Association

The BDA offer a number of awards to dietitians annually, and these are outlined in the *Dietetics Today* and in flyers circulated to members. It is always worth applying for BDA awards if they are appropriate to you. The Trustees will consider funding small projects. Details of when and how to apply are announced in *Dietetics Today*.

NHS Funding

Details of grants and requests for application for NHS funding are widely circulated to purchasers, providers and GP Fundholders for dissemination and may be advertised in the Guardian, Health Service Journal, British Medical Journal and Lancet. It may take a little detective work on your part. In addition, it may be possible to approach the Special Trustees of your hospital for funding.

Audit Funding

Ask your Audit Officer for advice.

Research Councils

The 3 main research councils that may be useful for nutrition funding are the Biotechnology and Biological Science Research Council (BBSRC), The Medical Research Council (MRC) and the Economic and Social Research Council (ESRC). All these are Government funded, and generally offer funding, primarily, for 3 year projects. Decisions to grant awards often take 6 months and the competition for funding from these sources often means that the majority of funds go to well established research teams. The application forms for these grants can be very daunting!

The councils also offer specific research initiatives which are advertised in the press. For example, the "Nation's Diet Initiative" funded by the ESRC was advertised in the press in 1991 and 1993. The Guardian Education section on Tuesdays is often the choice for such advertisements.

Government Departments

Both The Ministry of Agriculture, Fisheries and Food (MAFF) and The Department of Health (DoH) offer research funds in the nutrition area, but competition for both is very high. MAFF produces an annual report on its food research requirements, usually in October of each year, and this outlines all the areas it would like to fund, including work on applied nutrition. This document may be obtained directly from MAFF.

Research Charities

There are a large number of research charities who provide funds for research, and a complete listing of all UK registered charities is available from public libraries. Many have particular remits and you may find one which funds research in your area of the country, or aims to fund a particular candidate, and if you fulfil these requirements the subject area may be broad. The Association of Medical Research Charities produce a free annual publication outlining all charities in the medical area.

European Funding

Funds are available from the European Union but these mainly take the form of large collaborative projects between a number of institutions in different member states. Information may be available through Research Councils or Government Departments, but are probably only available to established research teams.

The Industry

Industry funding can be both "charitable" and for research purposes. A number of companies offer research funding, but many companies are willing to consider approaches from researchers if a topic is particularly relevant to the product or services. Support can be financial, but may take the form of equipment or consumables for use in a study. Individuals often have success obtaining travel grants from industry, particularly if they are local to a particular company.

Potential sponsors include food manufacturers, Trade Association bodies, supermarkets, baby milk/food companies and medical/pharmaceutical companies. Contact either the nutritionist, medical/scientific director or public relations department. Talk to representatives of companies that visit your work place if appropriate, and talk to company representatives at conferences and meetings. Care should be taken when seeking sponsorship. Check the guidelines of your department and hospital.

Studies Sponsored By The Healthcare Industry

If you are asked to take part in a study sponsored by a healthcare or nutritional company, ask if these are conducted according to procedures known as Good Clinical Practice (GCP). GCP procedures ensure that clinical research is conducted to the highest possible ethical standards and that valid, truthful data of high quality are generated. In particular, procedures for ensuring the protection of the rights of subjects participating in clinical studies are clearly defined and encompass the requirements for informed consent and study approval by an independent Research Ethics Committee which are enshrined in the Declaration of Helsinki.

Legislation and guidelines describing GCP procedures to be used in clinical studies of pharmaceutical products were introduced in USA in the late seventies and have become formalised in the European Union since July 1991 with the publication of the CPMP guidelines document "Good Clinical Practice for Trials on Medicinal Products in the European Community". GCP now represents a standard used by the entire pharmaceutical industry when conducting clinical studies.

Procedures for ensuring quality when carrying out clinical investigations of medical devices have also been in place since June 1993 which, while not specifically referred to as GCP, are to all intents and purposes, GCP. These procedures have been written as a European Standard (BS EN 540 1993 in English translation).

No written guidelines indicating quality standards or GCP exist for studies on clinical nutritional products. Nevertheless, some companies will require that all clinical research that it sponsors adheres to the high ethical standards demanded by GCP as well as to the rigorous procedures which ensure the validity and quality of research data.

WHY DO GRANT APPLICATIONS FAIL?

The 3 major reasons commonly given for application failures are:

1.   That the problem to be investigated is of insufficient importance or is unlikely to produce any new or useful information.

2.   That the proposed methods are unsuited to the stated objectives.

3.   That the investigator does not have adequate experience or training.

While you can work hard to remedy the first two of these, it is difficult for new researchers to get started since much emphasis is placed on the fact that previous projects have been successfully completed. As a new researcher, it is often best to affiliate yourself to someone either internally or externally, who can be named as principal researcher and has the experience required. Often their involvement may be limited, but they will add kudos and reliability to your proposal.

ADDRESSES

Biotechnology and Biological Science Research Council (BBSRC)
Polaris House, North Star Avenue, Swindon SN2 1UA. Tel: 01793 413200.

Chief Scientist Office, St. Andrew's House, Edinburgh EH1 3D9

Department of Health Nutrition Unit, Skipton House, 80 London Road, London SE1 6LW Tel: 0171 972 5298.

Economic and Social Research Council (ESRC) Polaris House, North Star Avenue, Swindon SNL 1UA. Tel: 01793 413200.

Medical Research Council (MRC), 20 Park Crescent, London, WIN 4AL.
Tel: 0171 636 5422.

Ministry of Agriculture, Fisheries and Food, Nobel House, 17, Smith Square, London SW1P 3JR.

The Association of Medical Research Charities, Tavistock House South, Entrance D, Tavistock Square, London WC1H 9LG. Tel: 0171 383 0490.

Methodology

METHODOLOGY

Once you have decided on the question you want to answer and you have conducted a literature review, you need to decide on your primary outcome measure and whether you will see a clinically significant difference between the old and the new treatments. If it is clinically significant you can then ask a statistician to calculate your sample size for you. If it is not clinically significant you probably need to redefine your question. For research to be useful it should be to the benefit of patients or service or there is not much point in doing it.

For example, using the question "Do overweight people with osteoarthritis lose more weight on a diet based on energy prescription rather than on a 1000 kcal diet?", the primary outcome measure we are interested in is the amount of weight lost. Using this same example, to calculate your sample size (i.e. how many patients you need to study) you need to decide how much greater the weight loss you expect to see on a diet based on energy prescription than on a 1000 kcal diet and whether you think the difference between the two diets will be clinically significant.

Only when you have an idea of the number of patients you need to study to answer the question, can you design your study, since, based on your sample size calculation, you may find that it will be impossible to find the number of patients you need or that the resources required to do the work are far greater than you have available.

Study design is the most important aspect of any research project, since the design is absolutely crucial to its success or failure. It is worth spending a long time, and consulting one or more experienced researchers, to ensure that you can actually do the study using the design you have created.

Going back to our example of weight loss in overweight people with osteoarthritis, you may decide you want to compare two groups: one group on a 1000kcal diet and the other on a prescribed energy level. However, to see a clinically significant difference in weight loss between the two groups, you need to study 100 people; 50 in each group. You know that you only see 70 people each year who would qualify, and not all would take part, so it would take 2 years to recruit patients.

Therefore, rather than comparing two groups of patients you might decide to ask 50 patients to consume two different energy levels using a crossover design (one energy level for one month followed by another energy level for one month) or do a retrospective review of a 1000 kcal diet in these patients and an interview in a group of 50 patients.

The sections which follow describe different methods of conducting research. The methods you consider will depend very much on the topic area you are researching, and in some cases it will be obvious from the start how the data may best be obtained. There are certain areas of methodology however, which require careful consideration, and it may be that you have to reconcile "best" methodology with limited research funds. You will have a good idea of potential methods of research for your subject based on the literature review you have conducted, and the starting point for information gathering on methods is always to review what has already been achieved.

Whatever size or scale of project you are attempting the methodological points are:

TYPES OF STUDIES

Cross-sectional studies

In these studies measurements on a subject are carried out at one point in time (snapshot). They attempt to assess the exposure of the sample to a number of factors and examine the association between these and the health or disease criteria of interest. Cross-sectional studies can be used to assess the usual diet of groups of individuals. They can be used to compare mean intakes between groups and can rank individuals according to intake. Cross-sectional studies are useful for measuring prevalence (e.g. number of people with and without diabetes who use artificial sweeteners) but not the cause of a disease (cannot tell from the above example whether having diabetes is likely to result in an increase use of artificial sweeteners or whether increased use of artificial sweeteners leads to diabetes).

Examples of cross-sectional studies include surveys of current knowledge, attitudes and dietary intake:

- A study examining insulin resistance, diabetes, risk markers for ischaemic heart disease and dietary intake in Asian and non-Asian men (Knight et al, 1992).
- The use of sweets as rewards in schools in one area (Burnett, 1994).
- The role of the dietitian in the management of malnutrition in chronic renal failure (Hartley et al, 1995).
- Comparing nutrition knowledge and attitudes in different groups such as consumers and health professionals (Rudat, 1992).

Calibration studies comparing one method with another are another form of cross-sectional study. Subjects are required to complete both forms of assessment and the results compared for each method. An example of a calibration study is comparing a food frequency questionnaire with weighed records (Thompson and Margetts, 1993).

Retrospective studies

Retrospective studies look back in time for associations between a disease or condition and potential risk factors. The most common form of retrospective study is a case-control study, where cases (with the disease or condition) and controls (without the disease or condition) are examined retrospectively to observe differences in exposure to the risk factors under investigation. For example:

*   examining the mental and motor development of children at 18 months of age and looking at maternal alcohol consumption before, during and after pregnancy to find out if there is a relationship (Forrest et al, 1991).
*   Comparing micronutrient intakes between cases with colorectal cancer and controls (Ferraroni et al, 1994).

Prospective

These studies follow a population group over time for a specified period, to monitor, for example, changes in variables (e.g. dietary intake, nutrient requirements, knowledge or attitudes) over time. Subjects may be selected because of some known exposure to a factor of interest. The follow-up allows for a comparison between exposure groups for example, between subjects developing heart disease and those free from the disease. Examples include:

*   Measuring dietary intake and blood lipids in healthy older men and women over a nine year period to see if any true age-related changes can be observed and examining the links between dietary intake and changes in plasma lipids in this age group (Garry et al, 1992).
*   Measuring the energy requirements and intake of a group of women throughout pregnancy to find out how they change and if there is a "gap" between intake and requirements (Van Raaij et al, 1987).

Intervention studies or clinical trials

Dietitians are very likely to be involved in these types of studies. These studies examine the effect or outcomes of an intervention or change. An "intervention" could be:

- A new treatment.
- Dietary change.
- Nutrition education/health promotion.
- Change in practice or service provision.
- Training.

Assessment of relevant factors may be made before and after the intervention and the changes measured. For example:

- Measuring the serum lipid response to dietary cholesterol in subjects stabilised on a low fat, high fibre diet (Edington et al, 1989).
- Assessing the benefits of health checks by practice nurses (Imperial Cancer Research Fund OXCHECK Study Group, 1995).
- Assessing the effect on attendance rates and treatment outcome in obese patients when given higher quality information prior to the first appointment at a dietetic clinic (MacQueen and Frost, 1995).
- Assessing the effect on dietary intake, food choice,shopping habits, eating together, meal planning and meal frequency of a dietary education programme to young mothers in a deprived inner city area (James et al, 1992).

Some studies attempt to do a rigorously controlled experiment in a population to prove cause and effect.

One way of doing this is for two groups to be randomly assigned to an intervention and non-intervention (or control) group. Both groups are monitored for pre-determined outcomes and comparisons made between them. For example, patients with recent acute myocardial infarction are randomly assigned to the control group (advice on a low fat diet) or to the intervention group (a low fat diet and additional advice to eat more "cardioprotective" foods). One year later outcomes such as mortality from cardiac disease, serum lipids and dietary compliance are measured to assess the effects of the additional advice (Singh et al, 1992).

For a summary of the types of study and the advantages and disadvantages of each, please refer to Table 3 and Figure 3.

Table 3. Advantages and Disadvantages of the Various Types of Study.

Type of Study	Some Advantages	Some Disadvantages
Cross-sectional	Easy to complete. Have control of the data. Can be quick. Provides baseline data. Highlight need for intervention. Can focus further research.	Results are descriptive and cannot provide answers to disease aetiology.
Retrospective	Simple and economical. Quick answers. Highly repeatable.	Dietary data difficult to collect retrospectively. Data may be inaccurate or incomplete.
Prospective	Data can be carefully controlled. May be able to investigate more than one hypothesis.	Costly. Very time consuming. Experience needed to set up and run the study. Follow up may be difficult if subjects leave the study or change their habits and lifestyle.
Intervention	Tests cause and effects. Subjects may benefit from intervention/treatment.	Difficult to change one component of the diet without altering others. Need to evaluate compliance of subjects. Controls may not receive a beneficial intervention.

Summary figure of types of studies. Figure 3.

	Past	Present	Future
Cross-sectional		X	
Case-control	X———————l		
Prospective		l————————————X	
Intervention		l————————————X	

Where X is the point of interest.
Adapted from Planning for Medical Research (Lowe,1993).

SUBJECT SELECTION

You will need to decide where your subjects will be recruited from. Will they be in-patients, out-patients (from which clinic), patients attending a particular health centre or a sample of the general population?

Inclusion/exclusion criteria

These will define who will be included and excluded from your study:

*   Volunteers/patients/population sample.
*   If patients, what diagnoses/medications are acceptable.
*   Gender, age.
*   Check your source to find out the size of the population available to study so that you can be sure of obtaining enough subjects in the available time frame.
*   Decide on your inclusion/exclusion criteria remembering that you need to be able to recruit sufficient subjects.

Sampling

Large studies aim to collect findings which could be applied to all individuals in a particular area, population or age group, and in this case the sampling must be random, so that every person in the population would have an equal chance of being selected. There are various methods of doing this. You may want to take the advice of your local epidemiologist based in public health or a statistician. (For sample size, see section on Statistics)

Response rates

The methodologies used in your study may affect the response rates for participation and completion. It is largely believed that response rates tend to decrease with increasing complexity of the survey method. Thus, response rates are likely to be lowered if subjects are required to complete methods which are demanding and impinge on their own time. A high response rate (90%) should always be aimed for. A low response rate or a high proportion of subjects not completing the study may result in an unrepresentative study sample and hence the results may not give a true picture of the real situation. Those subjects taking part may differ from those not taking part.

DATA COLLECTION METHODS

Qualitative data collection

Qualitative methods of data collection often form the basis of initial research procedures, and aim to collect descriptive information. Qualitative data collection may take a number of forms but often involves in-depth interviews or group interviews (focus groups). Qualitative research is by definition "open-ended" and often involves use of a semi-structured interview or observation form. It is common practice to tape interviews for later transcription. Interviewers need to be trained, experienced and familiar with the subject area. Care is needed in interpretation but this type of data collection can provide vital background information and new leads and ideas when trying to answer complex questions. It is useful for gathering information from "hard to reach" subject groups. There are many publications on the methodology and analysis in the social sciences literature.

Examples include:

- Studying schoolchildren's food preferences, eating behaviour and food choices using a combination of focus groups and observational techniques (Ross, 1995).
- Holding discussion groups with meal providers in Scotland to explore issues affecting fruit and vegetable consumption (Marshall et al, 1995).
- Interviewing local implementors of a national healthy eating campaign to find out their perspective of the campaign (Velleman and Oxford, 1994).

Quantitative data collection

There are many ways in which quantitative data can be collected in nutrition related projects, but they can be primarily grouped into:

a. data collected by questionnaire (see Section on Questionnaires).

b. data collected by dietary survey (Bingham, 1987; Fehily, 1983; Marr, 1971; Rohan and Potter, 1984).

c. clinical data and laboratory values.

Data collection forms

The forms you use for collecting your data should be designed so that they are user friendly. If you cannot collect your own data for any reason, someone else should be able to do it for you without having to read the protocol in detail.

Your data collection forms should have lots of white space, and you should not have to write down the information more than once.

You need to have a cover page with the title of the study and its number. The study title and its number should appear at the top of each subsequent page. On each page you should also have large clear boxes for patient's initials and study number. This information should be repeated on every page in case the pages get separated for any reason.

On the next page, in large clear boxes, put spaces for age, race, gender and any other demographic information you require.

The rest of your data collection sheets should be laid out clearly with, if possible, boxes for entering the data. The order of the data you collect should be the same as it is in your protocol, so that, if possible, you do not have to refer to your protocol - your data collection forms tell you what to do, and when to do it.

If possible, avoid asking open ended questions which requires free text in the answers, since this will be very difficult to analyse.

Finally, if you can design your forms so that they are automatically coded for entry into your computer database, so much the better. You will save yourself a lot of tedious work later!

TAKING MEASUREMENTS

Making measurements of any kind in a survey must be done with care, since it is easy to introduce bias. You may be taking anthropometric measurements, blood measurements, making measures of microbial safety or measuring clinical outcome for example, but in all cases a number of key points should always be considered. Your measurement method should be valid, reproducible and good quality control should be maintained.

Validity

This refers to whether a measure of exposure actually measures what it intends to measure, for example, whether a questionnaire designed to look at dietary knowledge with diabetes patients actually tells you the true level of knowledge. In some circumstances, particularly around the area of dietary intake, true diet cannot be measured. Therefore if a new method of assessing diet has been developed its validity against a measure of true diet cannot be made (Block, 1982). In this circumstance the new method is compared with a previously tested method "gold standard" with known accuracy. This is referred to as relative validity or concurrent validity.

Reproducibility

The reproducibility is concerned with whether the instrument or technique will produce the same result when administered repeatedly to an individual in the same circumstances.For example, hand dynameters should give the same result when repeated by the individual in similar conditions.

Quality control

Equipment should be carefully calibrated and regularly checked to ensure measurement are valid and reliable. Care should be taken with some measurements that they are not influenced by external factors, e.g. by the same time of day or the external temperature. Investigate thoroughly the measurements you intend to make and learn from the mistakes made by others. Ensure that local reference ranges for biochemistry are used. Different methodologies may give different results with the same analyses. These aspects should be discussed with senior laboratory staff. Standard forms should be used, if appropriate, to ensure good quality control.

PILOT STUDIES

A pilot study is a scaled down version of the larger investigation. Once you have decided on the method you want to use, it is essential to try it out on a small scale to see if it works. A pilot study will give you the opportunity to test your recruitment and data collection methods, and see if the overall organisation of the project runs smoothly.

A pilot study can also provide evidence that the goals of your research are realistic, and this can be very useful when applying for funding.

References

Bingham, S.A. (1987) The Dietary Assessment of Individuals: methods, accuracy, new techniques and recommendations. *Nutrition Abstracts and Reviews* (Series A) **57** 705-742.

Block, G. (1982) A Review of Validation of Dietary Assessment Methods. *American Journal of Epidemiology* **115** (4) 492-505.

Burnett, C. (1994) The Use of Sweets as Rewards in Schools. *Journal of Human Nutrition and Dietetics* **7** (6) 441-446.

Edington, J.D., Geekie, M., Carter, R., Benfield, L., Ball, M., Mann, J. (1989) Serum lipid response to dietary cholesterol to subjects fed a low-fat, high fibre diet. *American Journal of Clinical Nutrition* **50** 58-62.

Fehily, A.M. (1983) Epidemiology for Nutritionists, 4 Survey Methods. *Human Nutrition: Applied Nutrition* **37A** 419-425.

Ferraroni, M., La Vecchia, C., D'Avanzo, B.D., Negri, E., Franceschi, S. De Carli,A. (1994) *British Journal of Cancer* **70** 1150-1155.

Forrest, F., Florey, Cdu V., Taylor, D., McPherson, F., Young J.A. (1991) Reported Social Alcohol Consumption During Pregnancy and Infants' Development at 18 months. *British Medical Journal* **303** 22-26.

Garry, P.J., Hunt, W.C., Koehler, K.M., Van Der Jagt, D.J., Vellar, B.J. (1992) Longitudinal Study of Dietary Intake and Plasma Lipids in Healthy Elderly Men and Women. *American Journal of Clinical Nutrition* **55** 682-688.

Hartley, G.H., Gilmour, E.R. and Goodship, T.H.J. (1995) The Dietitians' Role in the Management of Malnutrition on Chronic Renal Failure. **Journal of Human Nutrition and Dietetics** *8* (2) 101-104.

Imperial Cancer Research Fund OXCHECK Study Group (1995) Effectiveness of Health Checks Conducted by Nurses in Primary Health Care: Final Results of the OXCHECK Study. **British Medical Journal** **310** 1099-1104.

James, J., Brown, J., Douglas, M., Cox, J. and Stocker, S. (1992) Improving the Diet of Under Fives in a Deprived Inner City Practice. **Health Trends** *24* (4) 161-164.

Knight, T.M., Smith, Z., Whittles, A. et al. (1992) Insulin Resistance, Diabetes, and Risk Markers for Ischaemic Heart Disease in Asian Men and Non-Asian Men in Bradford. *British Heart Journal* **67** 343-350.

Lowe, D (1993) *Planning for Medical Research: A Practical Guide to Research Methods*. Astraglobe Ltd ISBN 09522839 0 5

MacQueen, C. and Frost, G. (1995) Does Higher Quality Information Improve the Attendance Rate or Treatment Outcome of Obese Patients? *Journal of Human Nutrition and Dietetics* **8** (2) 137-139.

Marr, J. (1971) Individual Dietary Surveys, Purposes and Methods. *World Review of Nutrition and Dietetics* **13** 105-164.

Marshall, D., Anderson, A., Lean, M., Foster, A. (1995) Eat Your Greens: The Scottish Consumers Perspective on Fruit and Vegetables. *Health Education Journal* **54** (2) 186-197.

Rohan. T.E and Potter, J.D. (1984) Retrospective Assessment of Dietary Intake. *American Journal of Epidemiology* **120** (6) 876 - 887.

Ross, S. (1995) Do I Really Have to Eat That?: A Qualitative Study of Schoolchildren's Food Choices and Preferences. *Health Education Journal* **54** (3) 312-321.

Rudat, K. (1992) MORI Research. Attitudes to Food, Health and Nutrition Messages Among Consumers and Health Professionals in *"Getting the Message Across - Nutrition and Communication"*, Proceedings of a Conference held 12th October 1992 Edited by Judy Buttriss, National Dairy Council.

Singh, R.B., Rastogi, S.S., Verma, R., Laxmi, B., Singh, R., Ghosh, S., Niaz, M.A. (1992) Randomised Controlled Trial of Cardioprotective Diet in Patients with Recent Acute Myocardial
Infarction: Results of One Year Follow Up. *British Medical Journal* **304** 1015-1019.

Thompson, R.L. & Margetts, B.M. (1993) Comparison of a Food Frequency Questionnaire With a 10-day Weighed Record in Cigarette Smokers. *International Journal of Epidemiology* **22** 824-833.

Van Raaij, J.M.A., Vermaat-Miederma, S.H., Schonk, C.M., Peek, M.E.M., Hautvast, J.G.A.J. (1987) Energy Requirements of Pregnancy in the Netherlands. *The Lancet* **24** 953-955.

Velleman, G. and Oxford, L. (1994) Issues in Implementing a National HEA Campaign at Local Level. *Health Education Journal* **53** (2) 182-193.

BIBLIOGRAPHY

Cameron, M.E. and Stavaren, W.A. (1988) *Manual on Methodology for Food Consumption Studies*. Oxford: Oxford Medical Publishers.

Graessle, L. and Kingsley, S. (1986) *Measuring Change, Making Changes - an approach to evaluation*. London: London Community Health Resource. (Considers ways of evaluating traditionally "hard to evaluate" community health projects.)

Howe, R. and Lewis, R. (1993) *A Student Guide to Research in Social Sciences*. Melbourne: Cambridge University Press. ISBN 0521 40888 1
(A step by step guide on how to undertake research which investigates various aspects of society using surveys, interviews, biographical research, content analysis and other method.)

Kohlmeier, L. (ed) (1991) *The Diet History Method*. London: Smith - Gordon and Co Ltd. ISBN I 85 463066 0 .

Marshall, C. and Gretchen B Rossman, G.B. (1995) *Designing Qualitative Research* (second edition) London: SAGE Publications. ISBN 08039 5249X.

Pocock, S.J. (1983) *Clinical Trials: A Practical Approach*. Chichester: Wiley. ISBN 0 47 190155 5.

The Journal of the American Dietetic Association in 1988 had a series of articles on research methodology :

Henry, H. (1988) Nutrition Education Research Project Example: An Experimental Design to Test the Effectiveness of Two Nutrition Education Protocols in Reducing Serum Cholesterol. *Journal of American Dietetic Association* **88** 1066-1069.

Laramee, S.H. (1988) Food Service Research Project Example: Survey of Patients' Entrèe Preferences. *Journal of the American Dietetic Association* **88** 1065-1066.

Monsen, E.R., Cheney, C.L., (1988) Research Methods in Nutrition and Dietetics: Design, Data Analysis, and Presentation. *Journal of the American Dietetic Association* **88** 1047-1065.

Sins, L.S.S., Simko, M.D. (1988) Applying Research Methods in Nutrition and Dietetics. Embodiment of the Profession's Backbone. *Journal of the American Dietetic Association* **88** 1045-1046.

The American Journal of Clinical Nutrition (1984) **59** (IS) is devoted to Dietary Assessment methods.

For information on retrospective assessments of dietary intake see:

Rohan, T.E. and Potter, J.D. (1984) Retrospective Assessment of Dietary Intake. *American Journal of Epidemiology* **120** (6) 876-887.

Some useful journals in addition to the usual Nutrition, Dietetic, Medical and Health Care journals are given below - ask your local medical or nursing libraries to help you locate copies.

Health Education Journal (ISSN 0017-8969) published by the HEA. Contains useful papers and 1995 issues have included a "Research Methodology" series (Volume **54** nos. 1-4).

Social Sciences in Health - International Journal of Research and Practice (ISSN 1352-4127). Includes papers on social science methodology for example: Thomas et al (1995) "Comparison of Focus Group and Individual Interview Methodology in Examining Patient Satisfaction with Nursing Care". *Social Sciences in Health* **1** (4) 206-220.

Journal of Nutrition Education. American journal produced by the Society for Nutrition Education. Crammed with research papers on nutrition education.

Designing a
Questionnaire

DESIGNING A QUESTIONNAIRE

Before starting to compile a questionnaire there are several points to consider.

What is the aim of the questionnaire? What is being measured?

You should have a clear idea why you are using the questionnaire and what variables you are trying to measure.

Has anyone else used a similar questionnaire ?

Do a literature search on your topic to identify any existing questionnaires. It is desirable to use an existing questionnaire for the following reasons:

- It has already been used and tested.
- It may have been evaluated (although validity in one setting does not imply validity when used under different conditions).
- Your data could be compared with other studies.
- It will speed up the questionnaire design as this can be quite time consuming.

What are the resources available ?

Don't attempt research which is beyond your resources - it is better to answer a simple question well. Make a list of the resources you have - number of people available to collect data, time and funds which are available. These need to be balanced with a desirable sample size (see Statistics section), method of administration of questionnaire and recruitment of subjects.

PRINCIPLES OF QUESTIONNAIRE DESIGN

General

Use language which is simple and unambiguous. Avoid technical jargon. The wording should avoid any suggestion that one particular answer is correct/preferred.

The questionnaire should require as little time and effort from the respondent as possible and in addition it should be easy to process.

The layout of the questionnaire is also important. The questions should be well presented, avoid putting too many questions on one page. The visual impact of the form is also important, pay attention to clear print and colour. The questionnaire should be labelled with the title of the study, respondent's study identification number (name if appropriate). These should be repeated at the top of each page.

If the questionnaire is to be administered more than once to each respondent, there should be space to write in the number of the questionnaire (e.g. 1 for baseline, 2 for second administration). You may also like to include some additional questions/information such as age,gender, address/telephone number and date of completion of the questionnaire.

The questions

Every question should have a purpose. Avoid asking questions which do not help answer the question as this makes the questionnaire unnecessarily long and cluttered. Each question should only contain one idea.

You may wish to include questions to confirm responses for important issues.

Order of questions

This needs careful thought. There should be a logical progression through the form which is easily followed. Questions are best arranged in sections. Sections are best arranged in order of importance of the information to the study, so that the most important data are collected when both the interviewer and respondent are fresh and least bored. Any sensitive questions are, however, probably best left to the end.

It should be clearly indicated whenever the completion of a section is dependent on the response to a previous question, and the starting point of the next section should be clearly identifiable. It is best to minimise the number of skips or jumps which can occur, since too many can be confusing and sections can be accidentally missed.

Types of questions

Open questions are used to search for information and the interviewer records the replies in a freely written form.

Closed questions responses are restricted to one (or more) of a specified list of possible answers. These should also include an "other" option and space to write details and don't know.

Closed questions are easy to process, but open are more detailed and provide in depth information. One possibility is to use open questions in the pilot study (preliminary stages) and use the answers to create a list of options for closed questions which can be used in the main study.

All possible answers should be covered.

The answers

There are various types of closed questions - dichotomous (yes/no), rating scale, alternative statements, or multiple choice. If we consider the following question relating to a dietary supplement.

Do you agree that this drink will help you gain weight?

1. Dichotomous

a. Yes/No.
This is the easiest type of answer but forces respondents to answer yes or no. This is useful if you wish to measure tendencies or leanings.

b. Yes/No/don't know.
This type of answer gives the respondent the opportunity to say don't know.

2. Use a scale

a. A commonly used scale is the Likert Scale, using a range of options from strongly agree to strongly disagree.

Do you agree that this drink will help you gain weight?

Please circle the answer which shows how you feel about this drink.			
Strongly agree	Agree	Disagree	Strongly disagree

A 4 point scale allows some discrimination between strongly held feelings and less strongly held feelings.

A 5 point scale allows a neutral option.

Please circle the answer which shows how you feel about this drink

Strongly agree	Agree	Neither agree or disagree	Disagree	Strongly disagree

You may also wish to include a don't know category.

b. Another scale often used is the **Semantic Differential Scale** (Charles Osgood). This is normally a 5 point scale with opposite concepts e.g. good/bad, unhelpful/helpful, nice/awful.

Do you think this drink will help you gain weight ?

Please circle the answer which shows how you feel about this drink.

Very helpful	Helpful	Not helpful or unhelpful	Not very helpful	Not at all helpful

c. The Visual Analogue Scale is similar to the Semantic Differential Scale but does not have set points. Subjects are asked to make a mark on a horizontal scale. The distance from the end of the scale to the mark can then be measured by a ruler.

Please put a mark on this line to indicate how useful you think this drink is in helping you gain weight.

Very helpful _____ Not at all helpful

3. Multiple choice questions

Multiple choice questions are useful for measuring knowledge (where this is a correct answer).
They are quick to complete and easy to interpret.

Please circle the answer which best describes the nutrient value of this drink.

A   High protein and high energy.
B   High fibre.
C   Neither high in protein and energy nor high in fibre.
D   Don't know.

4. Rank ordering

This can be used to indicate the order of importance.
An entire list can be ranked or the top three items given.

Please rank the following drinks in order of helpfulness in gaining weight from 1-3.
(1= most helpful, 3 = least helpful).

Drink A.
Drink B.
Drink C.

Coding

Record information in as much detail as possible. For example, for age it is best to record
date of birth and date of interview and then compute actual age. The next best alternative is
to record age of respondent in years for adults, months for young children and weeks for
infants and lastly to use predefined age groups e.g. 0-4, 5-9 years. Specify units where
appropriate e.g. kg for weight, cm for height. Also indicate number of digits of accuracy
e.g. height metres _._ _

With closed questions numerical codes should also be printed alongside the listed choice
of responses. For open questions these can be developed later. If data needs to be entered
onto a computer, the best option is to code all the information into boxes on the right hand
side of the form. Numerical codes should be developed for non-numerical variables e.g.
1male, 2 female.Use one box per digit. Avoid using 0 as in many software packages 0 =
missing / blank.

To minimise data handling errors, avoid transcribing data from one form to another. Some
software packages have a verification option by which data are entered twice, preferably
by two people and the differences are then compared.

Method of administration

1. Interviewer administered - the interviewer asks and records the responses to the questions. This can be carried out in person or over the telephone. It is possible to clarify any confusion over what a question means. However, interviewing subjects is very time consuming and may not be practical for surveys with a large number of subjects, although the response rate may be better than that for self-administered questionnaires, particularly if they are sent by post.

2. Self-administered - a form is handed/posted to the respondent who completes the questionnaire. The instructions for completing the questionnaire may be explained by the interviewer or else written at the top of the questionnaire. In some circumstances it may be possible for questionnaires to be checked after completion to ensure all questions have been answered and also to clear up any ambiguities or problems the respondent may have had in completing the questionnaire.

The advantages and disadvantages of using interviewer administered and self-administered questionnaires are shown in Table 4 below.

Using a self-administered questionnaire compared with interviewer administered questionnaires there is less control over the completion of the questionnaire, response rates tend to be lower, questions may be misinterpreted or missed and it is also possible that other people may fill in the questionnaire. However if the sample size is very large a self-administered questionnaire is more cost effective and practical and there is no interviewer bias.

Table 4. Advantages and Disadvantages of Questionnaires.

	Interviewer-administered	Self-administered
Advantages	Can ask more complex questions. Higher responseto questionnaire.	Less time consuming for interviewer. Does not require skilled interviewers. Less costly. No interviewer bias. Large sample size. Respondents complete at own speed.
Disadvantages	More time consuming and expensive. Interviewer bias. Subject may answer in a way they think they are expected to. Trained and paid interviewers. Less questionnaires can be completed in same time. Smaller sample size	Response to mail questionnaires tends to be low. Biased sample may not represent population as a whole. Questions misinterpreted or missed Other people may fill in questionnaire Literacy More difficult to verify questions with respondent.

Suggestions

A covering letter should accompany every questionnaire. Explain who you are and why the research is being carried out and also the benefits of taking part to the respondent. Confidentiality should be ensured.

Thank the respondent for taking time to complete the questionnaire.

Evaluation of the questionnaire

Questionnaires should be subject to two forms of evaluation:

1. Pretesting - is an essential part of questionnaire design. Circulate drafts to colleagues, friends, relatives and ask for comments and criticisms. Redraft the form and repeat the process asking your advisers to try to answer the questions. This involves administration of the drafts of the questionnaire to samples of subjects similar to those to be studied. Its purpose is to identify questions that are poorly understood, ambiguous, or which evoke a hostile or other undesirable responses. Pretests should be carried out in the way that the questionnaire will be finally administered. This is particularly important for self-completed questionnaires as there will be no one around to help complete the questionnaire. Multiple pretests will usually be necessary before the final form of the questionnaire is obtained.

2. Pilot - select a small sample (not necessarily at random) of your target population and evaluate the responses. Each pilot subject can be handed a questionnaire and asked to complete it, whilst you are on hand to answer any problems the respondent has with its completion. You can then go through the answers of each question with the respondent to try and understand the meaning that he/she has attached to each question. If possible take several other people along to do this.

Assessment of validity and reliability - independent, valid measures of the variables will be necessary. Validation is usually difficult, often expensive, and sometimes impossible. It is often undertaken as a preliminary step with a sample of subjects. Reliability can be measured by repeating the administration of the questionnaire in a small group of respondents and comparing the responses.

Existing questionnaires may not be transferable from one group to another e.g. a questionnaire developed in adults cannot necessarily be used for children. Questionnaires which have been modified or used in different situations from which they were intended should be re-examined for reliability and validity.

Interviewer training

Interviewer training ensures that they are properly selected, briefed, and trained: they will make or break the project. Institute quality control: this means that you must check as many of the completed forms as you can personally and draw attention to the problems. Try to achieve a high response rate. Send out a reminder along with a second copy of the questionnaire.

BIBLIOGRAPHY

Hoinville, G., Jowell, R. and Associates (1985). *Survey Research Practice*, Gower Publishing ISBN O 56605 1567.

Oppenheim, A.N (1992). *Questionnaire Design, Interviewing and Attitude Measurement*. London. pp 303. Printer Publishers ISBN 1 85567 0445 (pbk).

FURTHER READING

Bailey, D. M. (1991) *Research For Health Professionals, A Practical Guide*. Philadelphia: F A Davis Company.

Leedy, P. (1989) *Practical Research Planning and Design*. New York: Macmillan Publishing Company.

Stewart, M. (ed) (1992) *Tools For Primary Care Research*. London: Sage.

Stone, D. H. (1993) *Design a Questionnaire*. British Medical Journal **307**: 1264-1266.

Ethical Approval

ETHICAL APPROVAL

What are ethical committees ?

The majority of ethical committees are Local Research Ethical Committees (LREC) which are organised on a health district basis as independent bodies to advise on the ethics of proposed research projects which will involve human subjects and take place broadly within the NHS.

They usually have about 8 - 12 members who should be of both sexes and from a wide range of age groups with a broad range of expertise. They will include at least two lay members, hospital medical staff, GPs and nursing staff, as well as other health professionals. LREC members act in a voluntary capacity and as individuals, not as representatives of their profession or employer.

Universities and other research institutes usually have their ethics committees, or a joint arrangement with an LREC. Research involving NHS resources as well may need to go to both committees.

Multicentre studies need to be examined by all the relevant LRECs even if a central committee has given approval already. Approval by an ethical committee is no guarantee of approval by all.

What sort of research needs ethical committee approval ?

If your project involves any of the following you may need ethical approval:

* The collection of confidential or personal information.
* Video or audio taping.
* Observation of subjects.
* The collection of tissue of any kind (including blood).
* Any deception.
* Any invasive procedures.
* Dealings with children.
* Dealings with anyone not able to give consent.
* Any procedure which might cause distress, even inadvertently.
* Dealing with anyone who might feel unable to decline to take part.
* Any other ethical issue.

An LREC must be consulted about any research proposal involving:

- NHS patients (i.e. subjects recruited by virtue of their past or present treatment by the NHS) including those treated under contracts with private sector providers.
- Access to the records of past or present NHS patients.
- The use of, or potential access to, NHS premises or resources.

What do ethical committees consider ?

The main responsibility of an LREC is to protect research subjects from harm and protect their rights without impeding the progress of valid research. For most studies, ethical committees need to include assessment of:

- The adequacy of the research design, organisation and resource arrangements (it is not ethical to use research subjects or NHS resources for research which is so poorly planned it is unlikely to contribute to an increase in knowledge).
- Risks or inconveniences to the subjects versus the benefits of the research (either to the subjects or expected collective benefits). The committee will look at how inconveniences or hazards are to be minimised or managed once they occur. Proper procedures for obtaining informed consent from the subjects are to be followed. Subjects have sufficient information (verbal and written) and time to give informed consent. This includes ensuring that subjects are not put under any pressure to participate against their will.

Getting the most out of encounters with ethical committees

Taking your research proposal before an ethical committee often seems daunting. Try and see it as an opportunity to check your research plans (regarding ethical issues) rather than as an obstacle to be overcome. The ethical committee is there to help you overcome any ethical problems (e.g. with obtaining informed consent without biasing your sample) and you may even get some useful suggestions on improving the study design, although a lot will depend on the individual committee methods of working. It is important to include planning for ethical approval at the start of the research planning process. Meetings in some areas may be only held quarterly.

How to apply for ethical approval

- Early in your research planning, find out from the Secretary or the Chair of the committee when the committee meets, how you should submit your research proposal and by what date, and how to obtain any forms you may need.
- If you are not sure if you need ethical approval it may be a good idea to contact the Chair or a member of the committee for advice.
- Submit your proposal in the format required and by the deadline given.

Many ethical committees use proformas and may issue guidance notes. Read these carefully and follow the instructions. Proposals should be typed. Write concisely, in plain English, avoiding jargon and remembering that many of the committee members will not have experience of your field or the methodology you are using.

Things to make particularly clear are:

- The aim of the research.
- The methods you will use.
- Details of proposed sample size, time-scale, resources needed and where these will come from.
- Criteria for selection of subjects.
- Sources of funding, inducements to yourself or the subjects etc.
- Actual or potential inconveniences or hazards to the subject (e.g. extra visits to hospital, time to fill in questionnaire, extra venepuncture etc.) and any plans to minimise or deal with these.
- How you will be addressing the issue of informed consent.(need definition of informed consent.)
- Copies of any subject information sheet and consent form.

If you are invited to attend the ethical committee meeting then go. This can be a great time-saver as it gives you the opportunity to clarify any points committee members do not understand and to discuss any unresolved ethical issues with the committee who should be able to help. If there are any aspects of your submission the committee are not clear about, and you are not there, your application may be deferred until the next meeting or you may be asked to resubmit, both of which delay getting started!

FURTHER READING ON ETHICAL ISSUES

Research on Healthy Volunteers 1986.

Research Involving Patients 1990.

Both Reports of the Royal College of Physicians of London, 11 St Andrews Place, London NW1 4LE.

FURTHER INFORMATION ON THE PRACTICE OF ETHICS COMMITTEE

Department of Health (1991) *Local Research Ethical Committees*, HSGC (91) 5 DoH London: HMSO.

Department of Health (1994) *Standards for Local Research Ethics Committee - A Framework for Ethical Review* DoH London: HMSO.

Report of the Royal College of Physicians (1990) *Guidelines on the Practice of Ethics Committees in Medical Research Involving Human Subjects* Second Edition

Statistics

STATISTICS

If there is one chapter in this publication that is tempting to skip it is possibly this one. However, it is also probably the most important since any study that does not have a good statistical basis is almost certainly a waste of time. For the most part statistics is the application of logic and simple common-sense and it need not necessarily involve lots of incomprehensible mathematics.

The first rule is if you are unsure, get help. Statisticians are relatively rare and often very busy people. Therefore if you need help it is best to go with a formulated plan and at least a draft study protocol. Always ask advice before you begin collecting data. The best help a statistician can give you is on the design of the study not the analysis. If a study is well designed the statistical analysis should be relatively simple.

THE DESIGN OF A STUDY

In designing a study the first objective is to produce a clear stated purpose for the study. The aim should be as simple as possible and clearly understood. It is far better to be able to prove a very simple hypothesis than to design a very complex study with a multitude of objectives and then fail to obtain any clear answers.

When you have decided on the main aim of the study you will need to consider if the study is a simple survey to discover the characteristics of a particular population or a comparative study to compare the effects of two or possibly more treatments.

You will need to consider carefully what your target and sample populations are. For example, if you wish to find out the characteristics of all diabetics (the target population) then it might not be relevant to examine a sample of patients attending a diabetic out-patient clinic in one hospital since the type of diabetic patient attending hospital out-patient clinics might be different from those attending GP surgeries. Also diabetics attending one hospital might be different from those attending another hospital in a different part of the country. One has to consider therefore whether the intended sample population is truly representative of the target population and modify the aim of the study accordingly. If you are taking a random sample of patients attending an out-patient clinic then your study is only truly representative of the patients attending that clinic.

If you are carrying out a survey of hospital patients you may wish to have comparative data for the population at large. For example, if you wish to find out about the social characteristics of patients attending a hospital out-patient clinic, you could consider finding out similar information from the National Census for the general population of the area in which the hospital is located.

If you are carrying out a study to compare the effectiveness of two treatments then in the aim of the study you will need to carefully state the "principal efficacy variable" on which the outcome of the study will be based.

It is important to understand the concept of a "null hypothesis". It is generally accepted that there is no difference between two study groups unless it can be shown statistically that the probability of the two samples coming from the same population is reasonably small. Although there is nothing sacrosanct about a p-value of "0.05" this is the level of statistical significance which is usually accepted and implies that the probability of the two samples coming from the same population is less than 1 in 20.

DETERMINING THE SAMPLE SIZE

The next important consideration is to decide how large a sample you will need. There is no point in carrying out any project on a small number of patients when there is no hope of achieving statistical significance. It should also be realised that studies where it is hoped to show no difference between two treatments usually require more patients than studies where a fairly large difference is expected between the treatments. You cannot carry out a relatively small study and then assume that the two treatments are the same because there is no statistically significant difference.

Ideally, you should ask a statistician's advice on the sample size. In order to calculate a correct sample size for a study the statistician will require the following information.

•   Is the main efficacy variable a qualitative response (e.g. yes or no) or a quantitative variable (e.g. a continuous measurement such as change in body weight)?

•   If the study is to compare the responses to treatment on a simple yes/no (or success/failure) basis then you will need rough estimates of the expected response rate and the difference in response rates that you wish to detect. For example, overall you may expect a 50% response but wish to be able to detect a difference of 15% in the true response rates for the two treatments.

- If your main efficacy variable is a quantitative variable, you will need more information including an estimate of the standard deviation (or variance of the data), which might be obtained from a previous similar study or a published paper. If, for example, your variable is the change in body weight you will need some data on the spread of the changes in body weight that are likely to occur over the study period. You will also need to decide the difference between the two treatment groups that you wish to detect.

- Another consideration is the "statistical power" of the study. If, for example, you expect the true response rates in two groups of patients to be 50% and 75% respectively, then the sample size will depend on the statistical power of the study to detect a significance difference between the two samples. The greater the statistical power, the greater the chances of finding a statistically significant difference and the larger the sample size will need to be. Studies are usually designed with 80%, 90%, or 95% statistical power.

Remember that the smaller the difference between treatments that you wish to detect and the more accurate you wish the results to be, the larger the sample size will need to be.

QUESTIONNAIRE DESIGN

The next important step from a statistical point of view is to design a survey questionnaire or study case record form (CRF). The golden rules are:

- All the questions must be simple and very explicit.
- Do not ask unnecessary questions. Keep the questionnaire as short as possible.
- Decide if each question has a simple yes/no response, a categorical response (i.e. a defined number of possible categories) or is a continuous variable (e.g. height or weight).
- Try and avoid "don't know" or missing answers.
- Define the units for continuous variables.
- Design the questionnaire so that all the responses are recorded in boxes.
- Consider using tick boxes for yes/no and categorical responses.
- It is important to collect accurate baseline information on any factors which may affect the outcome of the study.
- If possible, pilot the questionnaire to test for any inaccuracies or at the very least ask colleagues to comment before finalising it.

DATA COLLECTION

The most reliable way to collect information for any research project is to do it yourself and not rely on either other people or patients themselves to collect the information. Response rates are much higher for personal interviews than for postal surveys and by collecting all the information yourself you can make sure that the questionnaires are accurately recorded. If you do need to ask colleagues or other people to complete the questionnaires, make sure you discuss it with them carefully before starting data collection to ensure that everybody interprets the questions in the same way and recognises the importance of completing the questionnaire as accurately as possible.

Nowadays, for most studies, questionnaires are entered into a computer database or spreadsheet as soon as possible after the information has been collected. This enables further checks to be made on the data so that, if necessary, it can be corrected before the patient is unable to be followed-up. It is a good idea for two people to independently enter the data wherever possible. The two databases can then be compared to check for inaccuracies.

When comparing two treatments patients should be randomly assigned to either treatment, according to a previously drawn up schedule, so that there is no bias in the type of patient being assigned to either treatment. Wherever possible studies should be made "blind" (where the patient does not know which treatment they are receiving), or better still "double-blind" (where neither the patient nor investigator know which treatment the patient is receiving).

ANALYSING THE DATA

It is emphasised again, that if a study has been carefully designed with a relatively simple objective in mind and the data carefully collected, any statistical analysis should be relatively simple.

Many computer software packages produce simple statistical analyses. It is probably best to begin by tabulating the results for each of the variables recorded in the study (by treatment group if it is a comparative study). The frequencies (numbers of patients for each category) should be tabulated for all categorical variables; and the numbers of observations (N), means, and standard deviations (S.D.) for each continuous variable.

It can also be a good idea to produce histograms for the continuous variables, since many statistical tests are dependent on the data being "normally" distributed. If the data are normally distributed then the histogram will be reasonably symmetrical and look "bell shaped". Variables such as height and body weight are usually normally distributed, but data such as lengths of stay in hospital are not, since there is a tendency for the distribution to be skewed towards the bottom end, with large numbers of patients having short stays and a small number of patients having very long stays. In such cases one must either "transform" the data by analysing the logarithms, for example, or use a "non-parametric test" where the values are simply placed in rank order so that the underlying distribution is not important.

STATISTICAL TESTS

When you have simply tabulated all the responses, it would be a good time to discuss the results with a statistician and seek advice on the statistical tests you should use. A few simple tests are illustrated in Figure 4.

	Number of Comparative Groups		
Type of Data	One	Two	Three or more
Categorical	Sign test	Chi-square Test	Chi-square Test
Parametric (normaldistribution)	Paired-Comparison t-test	Two Sample t-test	One-Way Analysis ofVariance
Non-parametric	Wilcoxon Signed Rank Sum Test	Mann-Whitney "U" Test	Kruskal-Wallis Test

The Sign Test is a very simple test for use when there is a single group of patients. For example, if there are 20 patients of which 12 improved, five remained the same, and three became worse during the course of a study, then one could use the sign test to determine whether the results could have occurred by random chance without the treatment having any true positive or negative effect.

The Paired Comparison t-test is used in a single group of patients. For example, one could calculate the changes in body weight for individual patients and then use the test to examine whether the mean change in body weight for the group of patients was statistically significantly different from zero.

The Wilcoxon Signed Rank Sum Test is used to examine the changes in a parameter for a single group of patients when the data are not normally distributed, for example, the areas of leg ulcers (although in this case it might be possible to consider the square roots of the areas and use a paired comparison t-test). The signed rank sum test considers the overall rank orders of all the values regardless of whether they were positive (increases) or negative (decreases). It then compares the sums of the ranks for the positive and negative values.

The Chi-Square Test is used to compare two or more groups of patients with categorical data. For example, one could compare the numbers of males and females in two treatment groups using a 2 x 2 chi-square test. If there were three categories and three treatment groups then you would use a 3 x 3 chi-square test in order to determine whether all three treatment groups could have come from the same overall population.

The Two Sample t-test is used to compare the mean values for two treatment groups, when the data can be considered to be reasonably normally distributed. It should be noted that in many studies it is better to compare the mean changes in values from baseline rather than simply test whether the absolute values are different at the end of the study, since the changes will usually be less variable between patients.

The One-Way Analysis of Variance is the general case of a two sample t-test when there are three or more treatment groups. The one-way analysis of variance tests to see if all the treatment groups could be considered to have come from the same population. If the result is not statistically significant, there is no evidence of any difference between the treatment groups. However, if there is a significant difference then one should test the various pairs of treatments to determine where the main differences lie.

The Mann-Whitney U Test (or the almost identical Wilcoxon Rank Sum and Kendall's S tests) is the non-parametric equivalent of the two-sample t-test and could therefore be used to compare the changes in the areas of leg ulcers in two treatment groups. It works by calculating the rank orders of all the values and then comparing the sums of the ranks for the two treatment groups.

The Kruskal-Wallis Test is the non-parametric equivalent of the one-way analysis of variance.

95% Confidence Intervals are very useful to quote for the differences between treatment groups. For example, the mean changes in body weight might be 3.2 kg for treatment A and 1.9 kg for treatment B. Then instead of just quoting the difference as 1.3 kg you could also calculate the 95% confidence interval for this difference which might be say -0.5 kg to 3.1 kg. One would then be 95% confident that the real difference in the mean values lies within the range -0.5 kg (implying that the mean increase in body weight might be 0.5 kg greater with treatment B) to +3.1 kg (implying that the mean increase in body weight might be as much as 3.1 kg greater with treatment A).

Page 76

PRESENTATION OF RESULTS

Finally, when you have carefully tabulated all your results and carried out all your statistical tests the best way to get conclusions across is to present your data graphically using one of the many computer software packages that are now available.

The main types of graph are:

Pie Charts can be used to present simple categorical data such as the ethnic origin of a group of patients. If there are two treatment groups then two pie charts could be used alongside one another.

Histograms are used to present the frequencies of continuous variables by categorising them into intervals. For example ages could be presented in a histogram using 10 year intervals, 0 to 9 years, 10 to 19 years, 20 to 29 years, etc. Histograms are very useful in deciding whether data are reasonably normally distributed.

Scatter Diagrams are used to plot one variable against another. For example, one could plot age on the x-axis against length of stay in hospital on the y-axis. Most computer graphics packages will then fit a "trend line" (or the line of best fit) through the data so one can establish whether there is a relationship between the two variables. It is also possible to plot two such lines on the same graph in order to examine whether the overall trends for two treatment groups are similar.

Bar Charts can be used in similar circumstances to pie charts and are particularly useful when there are more than four or five categories. Multiple bar charts can be used instead of two pie charts to compare the numbers of patients in each of several categories for two or more treatment groups. Bar charts should not be confused with histograms.

Line Charts are particularly useful in plotting mean values over time. Hence you could compare the mean body weights, measured at weekly intervals for two treatment groups. Line charts plot the mean values for each week on a graph and then join up the values for consecutive weeks with straight lines (as opposed to a trend line which fits the best single straight line through all the points). It is often better to plot the changes from the baseline in variables such as body weight, rather than the absolute values, since both treatment groups will start from the same zero value at the start of the study.

BIBLIOGRAPHY

Altman, D.G.,(1991) *Practical Statistics for Medical Research*. London: Chapman, Hall. ISBN 0 412 27630 5.

Campbell, M. and Machin, D. (1993) *Medical Statistics, A Common Sense Approach*. Second Edition Chichester: Wiley. ISBN 0 471 93764 0.

Hannagan, T.N. (1987) *Lecture Notes on Medical Statistics*. Second Edition. Oxford: Macmillan Press Ltd. ISBN 0 63 201813 5.

Kahn, H.A. and Sempos, C.T. (1983) *Statistical Methods in Epidemiology*. New York: Oxford University Press. ISBN 0 19 505751 1.

Kirkwood, B.R. (1988) *Essentials of Medical Statistics*. Oxford: Blackwell Scientific Publications. ISBN 0 471 93764 0.

Swinscow, T.D.V. ('1993) *Statistics at Square One*. Great Britain: British Medical Journal Publications. ISBN 0729 01753.

Writing a Paper for Publication in a Journal

WRITING A PAPER FOR PUBLICATION IN A JOURNAL

Why publish ?

By publishing your work you make your research available to a wider audience that will include other medical professions apart from dietitians. For personal development, there is a great amount of satisfaction seeing your name in print.

Which aspects are appropriate for publication ?

The aim of your paper may be to report preliminary or final results of a study. Alternatively methodological aspects of dietary assessment are also important to write up. These could include the development and/or the evaluation of a dietary method. Aspects of the effectiveness and efficiency of dietetic practice are also suitable for publication. A review of a particular topic, for example dietary habits of school children, may also be of interest.

Which journal ?

Select a journal that has an appropriate readership for your project. For example if your paper relates to dietetic practice it should be submitted to a journal dietitians read. Most journals have an editorial policy on the types of papers they accept and this should be found under the Instructions for Authors. Alternatively a glance through the journal should give you an idea of the types of papers published. When first submitting a paper it is best to aim high and try a highly regarded journal. If you are not successful you can always try another journal later, but do not send your manuscript to more than one journal at a time.

One commonly used indicator of journal status is its impact factor. The impact factor of a journal is a measure of the frequency with which the 'average' article in a particular journal is cited during a particular period. It is calculated by dividing the number of citation of the citable items published in a journal during the two previous years by the number of citable items published. Impact factors are calculated and published annually by the Institute of Scientific Information (ISI). Generally, an increasing impact factor is an indicator of a journal of increasing status. The BDA journal, *Journal of Human Nutrition & Dietetics* for example, has more than doubled its impact factor in four years from 0.205 to 0.519.

When should the paper be written ?

Writing papers can be time consuming, as well as a daunting prospect. The task can be made easier if you have a good research protocol as this can be used as a starting point. The background and methods sections can be drafted while data are being collected.

HOW TO WRITE THE PAPER

Once you have decided which journal to submit your paper to, obtain the latest version of Instructions for Authors. These are usually published in the journal and often can be found in the first issue of each volume. For example, Instructions for Authors in the Journal of Human Nutrition and Dietetics can be found at the end of the first issue of each volume. Journals not only accept full papers but may also accept letters to the editor, reviews and short reports that present preliminary results or case-studies and are usually subject to word and table limits.

Instructions to authors guidelines

These should be read carefully. They indicate number of copies required and give details on line spacing, margin widths etc. There may also be a word limit for full papers (i.e. 2500 - 4000 words for Journal of Human Nutrition and Dietetics). The instructions may also give guidelines on the statistical treatment of results, nomenclature of vitamins, fatty acids and lipids and chemical formulae.

It may also be necessary if experimental work on human subjects was performed to include a statement that ethical approval was granted. A letter from the ethical committee may also be required.

Before writing the paper it is best to do a further literature search in addition to the one completed when planning the project as further papers in your area of interest may have been published, especially if the study took a number of years. These papers may also be helpful to give you some guidance on the format and content of your paper.

Title page

In general this should include the title as well as a short running title for page headings, keywords or phrases to facilitate indexing, authors name(s) and name and address of the institution where the work was carried out.

Summary

This should be written once the paper is completed. The summary should be concise and include who the subjects were, methods used, main findings and main conclusions. Include the main points you wish to convey to the readers and make the summary sound interesting as many readers may only read the summary (there may be a word limit).

Introduction

This should include a brief background to your study, the question you were asking and why you carried out the study. The research question you are trying to answer should be clearly stated (see Writing a Protocol and Seeking Funding).

Subjects

Describe the subjects in terms of number, gender, age, source (e.g. general population, diabetic clinic), methods of sampling, recruitment, response rates, inclusion and exclusion criteria and any other relevant information (Nelson et al, 1993).

Methods

Indicate the design of your project (see Methodology section) and the methodologies used. Dietary assessment methods should be fully described in the paper, see "Checklist for the methods section of dietary investigations" (Nelson et al, 1993). Newly developed questionnaires may be published in full or in part as an appendix to your paper. It is also important to include qualitative research methods such as focus groups and group discussions as well as laboratory techniques and biochemical measures. All methods should be clearly explained in chronological order. Details of tests of validity and reliability of methods used should be included. Methods which seem well known and basic to you may not be to the readers therefore give appropriate details. Quote the most recent references if available. Indicate when the research was carried out and the time scale of the project.

Analysis of dietary data - if food intakes have been translated into nutrients indicate how this was carried out. For questionnaires, indicate how portion size was determined (used food models, average portion sizes). State the name and version of all software packages used. Also indicate which food composition tables and editions were used.

Statistical analyses - indicate which methods you have used, whether data have been transformed or adjusted and methods used. Give references where appropriate.

Results

The results section should be given concisely and refer to the tables and figures. Do not repeat details included in the tables but select the relevant points and summarise the information. Do not discuss your results at this point, just report your findings.

Tables and figures

These are normally placed at the end of the paper with each table or figure on a separate sheet. The approximate position of tables and figures should be indicated in the margin of the manuscript. They should be numbered and titled, and should be self-explanatory without having to refer to the text. Footnotes can be used to give definitions for abbreviations. Acceptable signs for footnotes will be found in the instructions for authors.

Discussion

First, briefly state your findings and compare your results with previous studies. Indicate the relevance of your findings. Discuss the value and limitations of the methodologies and sample of subjects you have used. Discuss any possible bias or limitation in your results.

Acknowledgements

This may include other co-workers who would have participated in the project but are not authors. Acknowledgement of secretarial support and source of funding for the project may be given.

References

The accepted form for references will be given in the Instructions for Authors. When referring to other authors' work the names of the authors should be quoted in the text, with full details given in the reference section.

Appendices

Further material for example, questionnaires may be appended.

Once the first draft is completed circulate it to any other authors, or anyone you think will give you constructive advice, for comments. The Research Committee has set up a Peer Review Service - for further details contact the BDA office. It is possible that it may take several versions of the paper before the final version is produced.

Proofs

These are sent to the authors to make sure the paper has been correctly set up in type and not so that new material may be added. Small alterations may be allowed but excessive alteration may be disallowed or made at the author's expense. The proofs should be very carefully scanned to detect typographical errors and compared with the original version of the paper. There is an accepted protocol for making corrections to proofs, which the journal should provide. Corrected proofs should be returned without delay.

Offprints

Some journals will supply free of charge a set number of offprints to the authors. Further copies can be purchased, an order form may be enclosed with the proofs.

What to do if your paper is returned for changes ?

Your paper will have been reviewed by referees and their comments should be returned to you. If upon receiving the comments you still wish your paper to be published try to address the comments. For comments you cannot address or you do not agree with, justify your response and then re-submit your paper.

What to do if your paper is rejected ?

If your paper is rejected you should receive a letter indicating the reasons why. It may be that the journal was not appropriate for your paper. If you still wish your paper to be published, make any adjustments necessary and submit your paper to another journal. Remember to first consult the Instructions for Authors for that journal.

REFERENCES

Nelson, M., Margetts, B.M. & Black, A. (1993) Letter to the Editor. *Journal of Human Nutrition and Dietetics* **6**, 79-83.

BIBLIOGRAPHY

Booth, V. *Writing a Scientific Paper*. (1974) London: The Biochemical Society.

Hall, G.M. (ed) (1995) *How to Write a Paper*. London: BMJ Publishing Group. ISBN 0 7279 0822 7

International Committee of Medical Journal Editors (1991) Uniform Requirements for Manuscripts Submitted to Bio-medical Journals. *British Medical Journal* **302** 338 - 41

O'Connor, M. and Woodford, F.P. (1978) *Writing Scientific Papers in English. An Else - Ciba Foundation Guide for Authors*, London: Pitman Medical.

Whimster, W.F. (1985) What the Critical Reader Looks for in an Original Article: A Guide for Writers. *In*: Hawkes, C. and Sargi,M. *Research. How to Plan, Speak and Write About It*. Berlin: Springe - Verlag pp 85 - 109.

Abstracts and Posters

ABSTRACTS AND POSTERS

AN ABSTRACT

Essentially an abstract should be a miniature paper - it should sum up the key points from your introduction, methods, results and conclusions. In other words a well written abstract should give the reader enough information to understand why you did your study, how you did it, what you found and your conclusions. Abstracts are used to summarise a study either at the beginning of a full research paper or for reviewers to select your work for presentation at a research or audit symposia in your field. Writing an abstract requires a considerable amount of thought and organisation. It is not just a matter of chopping bits out of a full paper! You must try to identify the most important points of what may be a very detailed and long study. If you are submitting an abstract to a meeting you must interest your reviewers sufficiently to want to hear more about your work.

The following should be borne in mind when writing an abstract:

Check the word limit for your abstract by checking the Instructions to Authors/Contributors depending on whether you are summarising information for a paper in a journal or are submitting your abstract to a meeting. Adhere rigidly to this word limit - this may take a considerable amount of refining.

Check the format required for your abstract. When submitting an abstract to a scientific meeting you are often required to use a pre-designed form and must adhere to detailed instructions on the font size and pitch setting of your word processor. Check how authors names should be given (usually initials plus surname rather than full Christian names), add addresses where required and ensure the title is underlined or in capitals as appropriate.

Structure. Some journals or meetings require a structured abstract, for example with titles such as "Aim", "Introduction", "Methods", "Results", "Conclusions" etc. Even when an abstract is not required to contain these titles essentially it should follow this format, using a new line or paragraph for each section. Where possible, look through old abstracts from the meeting or journal to which you are submitting to gain a good impression of what is required.

Write your abstract. The abstract should begin with the purpose of your study stated clearly and succinctly. A small amount of background information to your study can then be given. The style of study should then be outlined, for example was it randomised, prospective or retrospective, controlled or blind. A brief descriptions of the numbers, age, sex and important characteristics should be included e.g. "12 male and 14 female adult surgical patients were studied". The study should outline the basic procedures performed and methods used to analyse the data. It should then summarise the key results, emphasising any new or important aspects of the study and draw relevant conclusions. If appropriate, finish off with references.

Finally, check the length of your abstract and make adjustments as necessary. It is a good idea at this stage to give it to a non-specialist to read to see if they can understand the key points and findings of your study. Ensure there are no spelling mistakes and that it is clear and well laid out. Re-check any instructions on the format of your abstract, how many copies are required and the deadline for submission. When using a specific form, make a few copies to practice on before you use your original. Ensure that you have got the abstract absolutely right before printing or typing it onto the form. Don't forget to keep a copy for yourself!

A POSTER

Designing a poster is similar to writing an abstract in that the information must be succinct, interesting and clear. Essentially, you can use the wording and format from your abstract, but as you will generally have more space you can give more detail and can use more text.

Space is still limited so find out:

- The size of the board(s).
- Are they portrait or landscape?

The key thing to remember about poster presentations is that they should be visually appealing so don't include too much text and use plenty of tables, graphs and charts to illustrate your key results clearly. Use bullet points to summarise the aims of your study and conclusions. Remember that key messages of your study should be easily identified by people browsing round the poster section of a meeting, and not hidden somewhere in a long detailed section of prose. Key results are seen best if placed at the top right hand side of the poster.

Speak to your medical illustration department about the design of your poster, as many excellent graphical computer packages are available to give you very professional results.

Make sure that the text can be read at a distance. Check how the poster is to be attached to the board, Velcro, pins, tacks etc. Allow plenty of time to set up your poster. Check your own transportation details to avoid any wear and tear before you get to your destination. A poster tube may help with transit.

- Use simple, concise and plain English.
- Include a small amount of background material.
- Include a clear statement of the aims of the study.
- Your abstract or poster should cover the following points:

- What you wanted to do.
- What you did.
- What was discovered.

- Avoid using clichés and jargon.
- Use short words and sentences where possible.
- Link ideas.
- Read instructions to authors or contributors carefully.
- Make sure the appearance is neat and without spelling mistakes or corrections.
- Check references.

Good luck with your submissions !

Dissemination

DISSEMINATION

Dissemination means sharing and making your research or audit project known to others.

Why disseminate ?

We need to disseminate to fulfil the very reasons for carrying out research in the first place! Dissemination is an integral part of the research or audit process, and not just an appendage for occasional inclusion. Many dietitians do, however, find dissemination difficult. This section provides some ideas to help you.

When to disseminate ?

Most people think of dissemination as happening once their project is completed, but it can take place at any stage of the process. Some form of dissemination should be built into the protocol and an appropriate amount of time allocated to it. If this is not done then it is likely that you will complete the project and no-one else will get to know about it!!

What to disseminate ?

Even if the entire project isn't completed, you can disseminate and concentrate on the stages you have completed or are currently working on, and mention aspects yet to be carried out. Some dietitians are "put-off" if they feel the research hasn't gone as anticipated, for example, if they have obtained unexpected results, or the methods used have proved unsuitable or not worked. Don't be deterred! It could still contribute to greater understanding of a subject. It can also be very helpful for others to learn about problems, and approaches that may not have the desired impact just as much as so called success stories! **Remember no research is perfect!!**

Who to disseminate to ?

Depending on the nature of your project, various people will take an interest in it. This may be at a local, regional or national level - or even international! But don't always wait to be contacted about your project. You will have to take the initiative too and let people know about yourself and the work you are involved in.

People who may have an interest include:

- Departmental colleagues, other work colleagues, and managers.
- Audit department.
- Clinical and unit team meetings.
- Purchasers.
- Health education/promotion and community services.
- Universities and colleges of further education.
- Local community groups, voluntary organisations, and charities.
- Pharmaceutical companies.
- Companies manufacturing special dietary products.
- Food manufacturers and retailers.
- BDA Branches and BDA Specialist Group meetings.
- Government agencies e.g. Department of Health.
- The media; newspapers, magazines, radio, TV.
- Various local, regional, national and international societies and forums.
- Study participants/subjects.

How to disseminate ?

This will depend on the opportunities on offer. If you utilise a number of approaches you will reach a wider range of people. If you are collaborating in your research, ensure everyone is aware of each others activities. Some possibilities are given below with a few pointers for success.

ORAL PRESENTATIONS

The usual points for any successful presentation apply. In addition you should consider the following:

- Send abstracts in on time, if presenting at a conference (remember to put all the authors names on it).
- Ensure that slides/overheads are clear and not crammed with too much detail. Use medical photography or graphics departments if available.
- Check your brief carefully; i.e. both parties are agreed on what you are talking about, the length of time, how it will fit in with the other presentations and themes etc.
- Practice your presentation (with visual aids) in front of colleagues. The best colleagues are those who will give some constructive criticism.
- When presenting your findings to different groups you can emphasise different aspects of your work to meet the groups interest.

- Keep copies of your presentation transcript. This can be useful when planning other presentations.
- Learn by watching the presentation techniques or others.
- Mention co-authors and give any other appropriate acknowledgements in your presentation. Omission can seriously offend!

ARTICLES AND REPORTS

- Check exactly the audience you are writing for i.e. their knowledge of the area for research.
- Write clearly and succinctly.
- Use appropriate diagrams, graphs, and photographs.

Helpline

HELPLINE

Don't try to go it alone! It can be very helpful to discuss your research and audit projects at all stages; from formulation of your research question/hypothesis right through to writing papers for publication.

Why ?

Discussion provides an opportunity for:

- A constructive and critical overview of the project.
- Detailed review of individual stages; completed, in progress, or planned.
- Reflection on issues and problems of concern.
- Obtaining advice and new ideas.
- Extending your range of contacts, and networking.
- Increasing your confidence and gaining moral support.

How ?

This will depend on opportunities available e.g:

- Formal presentations at meetings, conferences.
- Seminars and workshops.
- Informal meetings and "chats".
- Providing written summaries or progress reports for comment.
- Use of telephone.

Who ?

Don't just sit and wait to be approached! People won't necessarily know what you're doing. Take the initiative and make contact.

Depending on the nature of your project various people will be interested (see section on Dissemination).

BDA RESEARCH COMMITTEE

This Committee has a remit to promote research and audit. Members comprise of dietitians with varied research interests and experience who work in different settings; universities and colleges, hospitals, community, management etc. With this range of perspectives the Committee is in a good position to support dietitians involved in research and audit. Committee members can be contacted either individually or via the BDA office in Birmingham.

Terms of reference

- To encourage Dietitians to undertake research and evaluation of practice and publish their findings.
- To encourage high standards of methodology across the whole range of research and evaluation of practice.
- To make available information on research projects in which Dietitians have been or are involved.
- To investigate and provide information on sources of funding for research.
- To provide help and advice on request to Dietitians involved in, or wishing to undertake research.
- To facilitate peer review of draft papers for Dietitians wishing to publish research findings.
- To liaise with other bodies on research matters as appropriate.
- To liaise with BDA specialist groups and interest groups and BDA committees on research matters.
- To promote actively the education and training of Dietitians in research methods.
- To raise awareness of ethical issues and COSHH requirements.

Some initiatives undertaken by the Committee include:

- Organising and maintaining the BDA Research and Audit Register.
- Publication and update of the "Computer Software" list.
- The BDA Research Award.
- Peer Review Service.
- A research strategy for the Association.

BDA RESEARCH INTEREST GROUP

This was formed in 1996 to support dietitians wishing to undertake research or evaluation of practice. Details on how to join may be obtained from The British Dietetic Association.

The aims of the group are:

- To inform and help all dietitians involved in research and evaluation of practice.
- To provide a Forum for discussion of ideas and dissemination of information on practical aspects of research.
- To work in close co-operation with the BDA Research Committee.

BDA WEB SITE

Launched in May 1997, the BDA's web site provides information for members and the general public, and links to other sites of interest. Visit the website at htpp://www.bda.uk.com

General Resources

GENERAL RESOURCES

USEFUL BOOKS ON "HOW TO DO" RESEARCH

Bell, J. (1993) *Doing Your Research Project: A Guide for First Time Researchers in Education and Social Science*. (Second Edition) Buckingham: Open University Press pp176. ISBN 0 335 19094 4.

Crombie, I.K. (1996) *The Pocket Guide to Critical Appraisal: A Handbook for Health Care Professionals*. London: BMJ Publishing Group.

French, S. (1993) *Practical Research: A Guide for Therapists*. Butterworth Heinemann.

Greenhalgh, T. (1997) *How to Read a Paper*. London: BMJ Publishing Group.

Howard, K. and Sharp, J.A. (1993) *The Management of a Student Research Project*. Aldershot: Gower pp 238 (A practical guide written for those intending to present research for examination for a higher degree but of use to others as it includes detailed information on selecting a research topic, planning, literature searching, analysing and gathering data, potential problems and writing up).

Lowe, D. (1993) *Planning for Medical Research: A Practical Guide to Research Methods*. Astraglobe Ltd 1993 ISBN 0 9522839 0 5.

Margetts, B. and Nelson, M. (1991) *Design Concepts in Nutritional Epidemiology*. Oxford Medical Publications, Oxford: Oxford University Press.

Monsen, E. R. (1991) *Research: Successful Approaches* The American Dietetic Association. (It includes sections on all aspects of nutrition and dietetics research.)

Phillips, E.M. and Pugh, D.S. (1995) *How to Get a PhD: A Handbook For Students and Their Supervisors*, pp 224. Open University Press ISBN 0335 192414 9. (A practical and realistic handbook/survival manual for those who are thinking of "going for it" or who are supervising research students.)

Polgar, S. and Thomas, S.A. (1991) *Introduction to Research in the Health Sciences* (Second Edition) Churchill Livingstone.

Willett, W. (1990) *Nutritional Epidemiology*. New York: Oxford University Press ISBN 019 504 501 7.

Open/Distance Learning
Resources

OPEN/DISTANCE LEARNING RESOURCES

The Open Learning Foundation has produced two useful units in its Healthcare Active Learning Series on Experimental Research. Each unit is intended to take 35 hours to complete. The work books are a useful resource in themselves and should be available from your medical/nursing library.

- Keeble, S.(1995) *Experimental Research I: An Introduction to Experimental Design*.The Open Learning Foundation, Churchill Livingstone, London pp 139, ISBN 0 8039 5249 X.

- Keeble, S.(1995) *Experimental Research 2: Conducting and Reporting Experimental Research*. The Open Learning Foundation, Churchill Livingstone, London pp 139 ISBN 0443 05271 9.

South Bank University's Distance Learning Unit offers "Research Awareness" Modules, which can be bought as books or undertaken as a distance learning course for CAT points and a diploma. More details from: Distance Learning Centre, South Bank University, South Bank Technopark, 90 London Road, London, SE1 6LN. Telephone 0171 815 8254. Fax 0171 815 7899.

The Centre for Medical Education in Dundee has developed a package *"Moving to Audit: An Education Package for the Professions Allied to Medicine"*. Further details are available from: The Postgraduate Office, Ninewells Hospital and Medical School, Dundee, Scotland, DD1 9SY.

The University of Leeds runs an "Introductory Course in Research Methods for the NHS Professions". It aims to introduce the basic skills required for the design, conduct, analysis and writing-up of a quantitative research project, Further details from: Dr David Owens (course organiser) or Mrs Allison Iredale (course secretary). Postgraduate Taught Courses in the School of Medicine, Worsley Medical and Dental Building, Leeds LS2 9JT. Telephone 0113 233 2729. Fax 0113 243 3719.

Many Universities with undergraduate nutrition and dietetic courses now hold postgraduate courses in health sciences.

Local Contacts/Notes